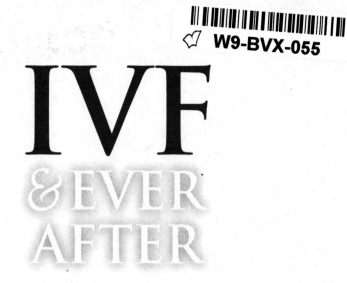

IVF & EVER AFTER

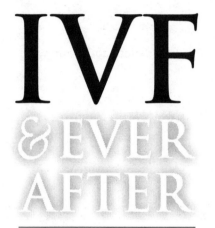

IVF & EVER AFTER

The emotional needs of families

Nichola Bedos

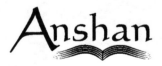

For Callum and Andrew

First published in the UK by
Anshan Ltd
in 2009

11a Little Mount Sion
Tunbridge Wells
Kent. TN1 1YS

Tel: +44 (0) 1892 557767
Fax: +44 (0) 1892 530358
E-mail: info@anshan.co.uk
www.anshan.co.uk

ISBN 978 1 848290 082

British Library Cataloguing in Publication Data
A catalogue record for this book is available from the British Library

Printed in

10 9 8 7 6 5 4 3 2 1

Contents

Forewords

Becoming a parent is a significant event in anyone's life, but when the path to parenthood is complicated by infertility and infertility treatment it may be even more emotionally difficult. The unfulfilled wish for a baby and the physical, emotional and financial demands of IVF are distressing experiences that can erode a couple's self-confidence and sense of well-being. Although the chance of having a baby with IVF is improving, most couples who pursue treatment will need several attempts to reach the goal of parenthood. When treatment is unsuccessful or when an IVF pregnancy miscarries, couples describe intense feelings of loss and sadness. Added to this are feelings of personal failure and doubts about whether the dream of a family will ever come true.

Those who persist with treatment and become parents feel extremely grateful that the treatment has worked and have high expectations of life with the new baby. But sometimes the transition to parenthood after IVF poses unexpected challenges. Anxiety about the ability to sustain and keep the baby alive, lack of confidence about the capacity to care for the baby, and feeding and settling difficulties are common after IVF.

While they are involved with the IVF program, couples have access to counselling to help them deal with the ups and downs of treatment. But, once a pregnancy is confirmed, there is little support and information available that meets the needs of couples who become parents after treatment. Nichola Bedos's *IVF & Ever After* is a thoughtful and insightful book that explores the emotional aspects of infertility, IVF treatment and parenting after IVF. It is a very welcome resource for health-care professionals and the growing group of couples who become parents after a long and difficult journey.

Dr Karin Hammarberg
Research Fellow, Key Centre for Women's Health in Society
The University of Melbourne

*

Welcoming a new baby into the world marks a new beginning for any parent, but for many couples experiencing infertility it becomes an even more significant milestone. The explosion in the number of IVF treatments performed in the last decade and the doubling of the success rate of IVF in the last twenty years herald a new generation of IVF families.

The medical technology that has enabled this process has had a profound effect on the lives of numerous families all over the world. While medico-legal, political and ethical dialogues continue to rage around it, IVF technology has paved the way for more than a million miracles to happen, opening doors to older parents, surrogacy and same-sex families.

The journey of every parent is unique and the experience of IVF is intrinsically individual. However, the psychological impact and emotional cost of the IVF process on couples cannot be underestimated. The need for psychological counselling is paramount in supporting their tumultuous emotional journeys. Optimally, psychological counselling must begin as soon as the diagnosis of infertility is made. The euphoria of a successful IVF treatment, resulting pregnancy and successful childbirth is more often accompanied by a myriad of complex emotions tinged by grief and loss. In the event of prematurity or medical challenges, the clinical diagnosis of post-natal depression compounds their emotional vulnerability.

In *IVF & Ever After*, Nichola Bedos, psychotherapist, has sensitively but candidly captured the unique psychological journey of families who parent the IVF child. This book is an essential tool for health professionals working with IVF families, those exploring IVF as an option and the general community to enhance their understanding and insight into the challenging journey of IVF parenting.

Lisiane LaTouche
Director of Social Work and Psychology, Tresillian, Sydney

Introduction

In 2006, some one million cycles of In-Vitro Fertilisation (IVF) were undertaken in more than 52 countries throughout the world. Almost 200,000 IVF babies were the result of this treatment. With new technology achieving success rates that were unthinkable even a decade ago and new practices making the process more affordable for ordinary families, IVF births are set to become a highly significant part of the world's fertility rate. Already, some countries such as Denmark boast a rate of almost four assisted conception births for every 100 births.

The technique's quiet beginnings belied its later success. Few people would remember 10 November 1977, even though this date heralded the beginning of the first 'miracle' baby, Louise Brown. On that day, her mother Lesley underwent implantation of a fertilised egg – which was to become the world's first IVF embryo to survive beyond a few weeks' gestation – into her womb. At that perilous stage, no one, not even the IVF pioneers themselves, had any idea that this procedure would mark the first IVF success. With great excitement, Louise was born by caesarean section on 25 July 1978. Three decades later, IVF has been used in the creation of three million babies.

As with all of the world's human-made miracles, media headlines have revealed the excitement and the scientific technique but little of the human side to this amazing story. Being the first miracle baby, Louise has endured much media attention. Interviews throughout her life to date have revealed a very sensible and practical person who has suffered the intrusion into her private life with dignity. What has never been described was the emotional roller-coaster ride experienced by Louise's parents. They lived through a nine-year struggle to become pregnant and the devastation of a diagnosis of blocked fallopian tubes, and finally experienced hope when Doctors Edwards and Steptoe offered them the opportunity of IVF treatment. There must have been anxiety throughout the pregnancy and feelings of absolute elation, combined with deep apprehension as the date of the birth neared.

How did IVF influence Louise's approach to becoming a mother herself? She gave birth to a son late in 2006. What will she tell her child when it comes time to discuss 'where babies come from'?

The science has made miracles happen. But there is a cost. The year 2003 marked an important turning point in IVF treatment. Research published then found that the use of this technique does impact upon the psychological well-being of both parents and child. Successful IVF treatment brings joy on a scale that is unimaginable to those who conceive without assistance, yet studies reveal this joy is also mixed with deep-seated anxiety. For truly informed consent to be obtained before couples undergo IVF treatment, they need to understand the factors that can affect their physical and *mental* health and how to access help to sensibly deal with these stresses.

Promising research by clinical teams around the world points the way to understanding the stress that IVF couples experience. It has been known for years that infertility can lead to anxiety and depression in both men and women and that it plays a role in some relationship breakdowns. A 2003 report published in the *Journal of Marriage and Family* indicated that involuntary childlessness poses a significant risk to women, even if those women go on later to have a child of their own through assisted means.[1]

Once a couple has been confirmed suitable for IVF, participation in treatment is a relief; however, partners often rate the technique itself as highly stressful, with women generally experiencing this stress to a greater degree than men. Women handle treatment stress quite differently to men: a 2006 study revealed that they seek support and talk about the difficulties, whereas men distance themselves or engage in problem-solving behaviour.[2] The stress can actually get in the way of IVF success because it reduces both sperm quality and the chance of an embryo developing inside the womb.

A pregnancy after IVF treatment produces excitement mixed with frequent periods of anxiety during the early months as the parents-to-be await the three-month point when the rate of miscarriage falls dramatically. Parents I have worked with report intense panic reactions to a twinge or spotting episode. They need calm, wise support to deal with these reactions.

IVF parents also benefit from good birth planning because the adoption of sensible strategies, which consider all available options, brings about healthier parent-baby relationships. Good preparation for birth is as vital to parents as intense training is to elite athletes. You come to the stress of the event with clarity of mind.

The stress may not end even though a healthy baby is born. Studies have shown that there are areas of parenting that couples using IVF can struggle with in the early years. A 2007 Dutch study[3] of five- to eight-year-old IVF children reported much more parental stress after IVF than after natural conception. An earlier study in Germany in 2004[4] suggested that IVF parents typically do not voice their negative feelings about parenting and may indeed have idealised views about parenting that are not realistic.

This book is intended to raise awareness of the emotional issues that can arise during treatment, pregnancy, birth and the years of parenting, and to provide simple, thoroughly researched strategies to address these issues. These strategies act to heal the damage infertility and stressful treatment can cause, leaving parents to raise their children with calm clear minds.

Today, humankind is so much better at scientifically achieving IVF success with healthy births, fewer multiples and fewer premature babies. We have embraced this amazing miracle technique and IVF treatment is now commonplace. It is time to focus on the emotional aspects of IVF. The miracle of life can then be properly enjoyed for a lifetime.

*

Many people helped to create *IVF & Ever After*. Thank you to Frank for being my sounding board and 'phrasing stylist', to my mother Diana for all her proofreading and for being the first person apart from me to tackle the book, and to all associated with Rockpool Publishing for the advice and encouragement to make the idea become a reality. Particular thanks must go to all the professionals who spoke to me and who contributed comments and research: there are a number of amazing people working with IVF families. I am also especially grateful to the wonderful families who have told their courageous stories, allowing me inside their homes and their lives to share the ups and downs of parenting with them. I have incorporated the experiences of many people from all over the world; however, names have been changed to preserve their identities, except when the family concerned has given me their express permission.

1

The Emotional Impact
of Infertility

*It was distressing for both of us to be constantly asked, 'Are you
pregnant yet?'*

Currently, around 15 per cent of all couples worldwide struggle with
infertility. Whilst this figure does not mean that all such couples will
be unable to conceive eventually, it does indicate a high level of stressful
'waiting' to fall pregnant that can affect all aspects of life. Even though we
now have the technology to work miracles for some couples, the emotional
consequences of infertility cannot simply be 'shrugged off', nor can couples
simply 'get over it', blindly rushing off to a private clinic to pay for
expensive and invasive infertility treatment. Those who have been
diagnosed with fertility problems require good psychological support to
explore the complexities of their feelings before IVF treatment can be
successfully attempted. Arriving at the door of an infertility clinic without
having reflected on the feelings evoked by a diagnosis of infertility can be
disastrous.

'No matter what the doctor offered us, the diagnosis of "infertility"
was there like a dark cloud hanging over us. I didn't feel science could ever
really overcome it. I felt a failure. It was my fault,' one woman explained.

She later went on to give birth to a healthy little girl, yet she still labels herself 'infertile'. In common with many other mothers, she has a sense of failure, of needing outside help and sometimes of thinking that the pregnancy and the baby somehow are not truly 'hers'. It is pervasive, damaging and it is a real threat to parents' and children's self-esteem. But it is treatable.

I started working with families with IVF babies in 2002. My counselling practice concentrates on treating families with young children, specialising in helping parents to parent in a more positive way.

At first, when I began working with an IVF family, I downplayed the importance of the manner of conception and treated the family very much in line with the conventional wisdom regarding parents who were experiencing anxiety and difficulty separating from their young child. Although I achieved some success with my normal repertoire of strategies, I found the family's pervasive anxiety about 'something being very wrong' hard to understand. It was only the following year that I came to understand the complexity of the issues IVF raises for prospective parents throughout the treatment process and during parenting. I came to see the tremendous impact IVF can have on the whole family, even extending to grandparents, aunts and uncles.

Treating a family who had not yet set foot inside the door of an IVF clinic startled me. Within weeks, I was questioning how the problems they faced could have arisen without a traumatic event taking place. The family was enormously emotional and irritable, which caused incessant arguments, particularly between mum and dad. There was a lot of anger from unresolved grief over a previous miscarriage. Family functioning was at an all-time low. The family's two children, who had been conceived naturally, were also exhibiting signs of behavioural disturbance. Although I am not suggesting all families are as traumatised as this one was, I have since found that many do exhibit similar symptoms of stress. At times, particularly during the phases when they are coming to terms with infertility, deciding to use IVF and the treatment itself, emotions arise that are simply too much for a couple to handle alone.

Even after this experience, I was not convinced there was any particular 'pattern' of need specific to IVF families. But several months later I began working with another IVF couple and their child. Again I perceived this pervasive fear of loss and the sense of danger that began before the IVF treatment process had commenced, together with the difficulty in separating for both parents and child. I began to sense there was something different about IVF families. I decided that, as a helping professional, I needed greater knowledge about the use of IVF as well as specific therapies to help the family to heal. I undertook research on the subject, finding a few studies that demonstrated heightened anxiety in couples undergoing the procedure. Again I discovered this same pervasive fear of loss and a sense of danger that began before the IVF treatment process had commenced, together with the difficulty in separating from each other for both parents and child. I began to sense there was something different about IVF families. As a helping professional, I felt that I needed to know the extent to which these problems were affecting my client families and whether such problems were being unearthed by other professionals working with IVF families.

I began by completing a small study of my own families in 2005. I conducted a simple analysis of the number of families with IVF children as a proportion of my total client base. Surprisingly, almost 20 per cent of my clients, twenty of the one hundred families working with me, had used IVF even though this may not have been the problem they originally presented with. In comparison, only 3 per cent of babies born in my country at the time were IVF babies. This study confirmed my suspicions that IVF families in my community were indeed needing help more often than non-IVF families.

The next piece of the IVF story came with research I undertook with the help of the Internet, discovering a number of well-respected studies into the stress and coping skills of IVF families as compared with non-IVF families. Evidence first surfaced in the late 1990s with a study in the journal, _Human Reproduction_ in 1998[1] contrasting parenting of IVF twins as compared to that of naturally conceived twins. Child behaviour in both groups was similar but IVF parents in this study reported far greater stress in their parenting than naturally conceiving parents. A further study in 1999[2] of parents with one-year-old twins conceived both naturally and with IVF revealed similar findings. IVF mothers particularly, reported greater parenting stress and relationship difficulties with their partners than mothers conceiving naturally. These mothers also felt less competent than their naturally conceiving peers.

My own findings were clearly being replicated elsewhere in the world. These findings motivated me to put together a treatment plan for helping IVF families in need, right from a diagnosis of infertility, throughout the IVF treatment process to the parenting of children born after treatment. The plan needed to be flexible enough to accommodate the vastly different situations families using IVF find themselves in, but it must always start with a recognition of the impact a diagnosis of infertility has on a couple.

Conception today

Our modern society leads us to believe a family of our own is always a choice we are able to make. Couples try to conceive a baby, believing it will only be a matter of time before a successful pregnancy is achieved and a healthy child is born. Advances in medical science have given the human race the sense that 'everything can be achieved eventually'.

We are bombarded with this 'we can do anything' philosophy. The media constantly reports stories about increasingly mature mothers giving birth. Many women feel they are more in control of their bodies than ever before and that age is no longer a barrier to having a career and a family.

Expectations are artificially raised.

But, with as many as one in six couples experiencing infertility, these expectations may be shattered. This can leave couples feeling isolated, 'different' and eventually like failures. No matter what follows, their self-esteem and psychological well-being suffer sizeable blows.

What I have found from working with IVF families is that these overwhelming feelings from the infertility diagnosis are often left unresolved. IVF clinics offer counselling, but this is focused on the IVF process itself — how to cope with it and what to expect — rather than on the circumstances that brought the couple to the clinics in the first place. Gynaecologists and fertility experts will usually explain the issues around the couple's problems from the medical points of view, but have little knowledge of what the psychological impacts may be. No one sits down with the couple, acknowledges their huge emotional stress and then tells them how to cope.

When IVF begins, the couple are often not mentally adjusted. Psychological work must begin as soon as an infertility diagnosis is made. For parents who have already given birth to an IVF child, this work can take place retrospectively to avoid unresolved grief affecting the parent-child bond.

The grieving process

The first and most common emotional reactions to a diagnosis of infertility are sadness and loss. The couple need to grieve about the fact that the normal vision of conception and parenthood will not be an option for them. This is an important reaction, not to be devalued or brushed aside, but it needs time and energy to accept.

The grief accompanying a diagnosis of infertility is complex. By this I mean that there are a number of different losses that couples must face. The infertility experts Doctors Aniruddha and Anjali Malpani describe these different losses in their book *How to Have a Baby: Overcoming*

Infertility. They include feelings of loss over potential children and their non-ability to pass genes on to the next generation. This puts a great strain on marriages, as couples wrestle with the feelings that life is now meaningless. Couples also experience loss of the experience of natural conception, pregnancy and birth.

Another loss that often goes unrecognised is the loss of privacy — and, indeed, ownership of their body for men and women, both of whom may have been through dozens of invasive tests to reach a diagnosis. Malpani and Malpani explain, with startling clarity, the sheer unnaturalness of the explorations involved, quoting one patient who felt she had donated her body to medical science. Daily temperature charts, blood tests, sperm tests and records of love-making can turn a previously cherished and satisfying aspect of life into one that is to be dreaded. All these feelings eat away at a person's self-esteem. These same feelings may again come to the fore after a pregnancy is achieved and a baby born.

To grieve means to experience deep and lasting sorrow. To grieve effectively does not have to mean shutting yourselves away for months or exploring the pain of infertility for days at a time. Grieving means that you recognise your emotions, that you acknowledge and try to understand them and that you express your sorrow in the way that suits you best.

The pioneer of our modern understanding of grief was a wonderful American woman, Elisabeth Kubler-Ross, whose work still shapes much of the professional help that is available to grieving people. Kubler-Ross described people passing through five stages during grieving; how quickly these stages occur depends very much on the person involved and the nature of the loss. You may also pass through some stages several times during the period of grieving.

Firstly, the loss is met with shock and a feeling of numbness. This is a chemical reaction in the brain designed to protect humans from feelings that are too overwhelming to comprehend. Parents often say they feel they are walking in mist for the first weeks after being told they could not conceive naturally. This is a stage that cannot be rushed and little can be done to 'clear the head'. What helps seems to be time to reflect and make sense of what has happened, the opportunity to talk to friends and family who can provide unconditional love, and the understanding of one partner for another. It is not uncommon for some people to deny the situation initially, rushing to book second or third medical opinions or searching the world for natural 'miracle' cures. Again, time will be the healer that eventually allows both partners to face up to the reality of the situation.

As the numbness wears off, it is usually replaced by anger: at the world for its harshness; at God if religion is a part of life; at a partner for being the one 'responsible' for the infertility, and at parents who have not had to go through this grief. For people not used to sudden anger, this can be a frightening time. This is the stage when sudden flashes of irritability can easily ignite into a full-blown fight for partners struggling to stay together on an emotional level. The anger may also be turned on well-meaning friends and family who offer up clichés as reassurance.

Anger need not be a negative emotion but one designed to help humans cope. If used wisely, anger can be a positive phase of healing. It may drive people to find a solution, to keep going despite disappointments and to avoid turning inwards into depression. The key to dealing with anger is to express it in harmless ways. Anger exercises, such as keeping a daily journal to chronicle your early feelings or writing an angry letter to friends with children or to someone who has hurt you (but not sending it), are invaluable. These are ways to let out all the pain and frustration being felt. It may be helpful to have a ritual letter-burning ceremony once the worst of the anger has passed.

The third phase of grief, according to Kubler-Ross, is bargaining. Bargaining may involve praying: 'If only I could overcome infertility,

I would be a better person.' Humans search for some reason that something bad has happened so they can find a way to put it right and, therefore, get rid of the pain. Again, this is a very normal way of dealing with a painful situation and is best helped by partners, friends and family simply listening rather than arguing that bargaining thoughts are not likely to work. This bargaining is just another step the brain takes on the road to making sense of loss.

The fourth stage, perhaps the longest to move through, is that of depression. As reality dawns, so partners experience the full force of their sadness, beginning to recognise that natural conception will never be theirs. Women may find themselves crying at odd times, unable to look at children playing in the street and deliberately avoiding pregnant friends. Men may experience low self-worth, impotence and feelings of the loss of their manhood. All of these feelings will be resolved in time if partners are allowed to cry, express sadness, talk about the dream child they will now not have and receive the support of others.

Finally, if the preceding four stages are navigated successfully, partners will reach Kubler-Ross's final stage of acceptance. This is not necessarily a happy and confident place but one in which partners feel more able to look at their situation realistically, to evaluate other options, such as assisted conception or adoption, or to decide to remain childless and pursue other meaningful goals.

Stuck in the grieving process

Even after the birth of a healthy baby, many IVF couples remain embedded in cycles of anger and depression, at times feeling worthless or feeling intensely and unrealistically angry with a friend who has reported conceiving 'first go'. There may also be difficulties appearing in the relationship because of the different coping styles men and women adopt in the face of great stress.

Most people become stuck in their grieving by avoiding the terrible sadness that acceptance brings or by holding someone else responsible. They may distance themselves from friends who have children, refuse to talk about their diagnosis or seek 'alternative therapies' in the hope of achieving 'miracle' cures. They may blame each other, God or their own continual bad luck.

In contrast, couples who move through their grief are those who face their infertility diagnosis head-on. They discuss their feelings together and with close friends. They acknowledge that infertility is a painful burden to bear at times. Most importantly, couples who successfully navigate infertility and its associated grief are those who can engage in problem-solving. They research the literature about infertility and use the internet to gain a greater understanding of the difficulties they face. They ask questions of the doctors they see. They review the options they may have and assess each one carefully, evaluating the 'pros' and 'cons', including the realistic costs involved. They remain focused on generating ideas, suggestions and new paths to take.

Special circumstances

Grief does not always depend on how bad the loss is, as measured on a fixed scale. Some people may view the loss of natural conception as the worst event to happen in their lives; another couple may be sad but less affected by grief. Both reactions are entirely normal. However, there are certain circumstances for couples suffering infertility that may complicate and prolong grief.

A number of couples requesting my professional assistance have faced the prospect of using IVF as their only means of conceiving a healthy child, not because either is infertile but because one or both parents carry a genetic abnormality, which may be passed on to a naturally conceived child. Genetic abnormalities can include extra genes, deletion of certain parts of a gene or insertion of extra genetic material into a gene. These abnormalities can lead to failure of the embryo to implant, failure to develop normally or to a baby being born with a genetically determined disorder such as cystic fibrosis. These parents have losses to grieve, but often they also experience guilt at being the carrier of a gene that could hurt an unborn child.

This may be complicated if the couple already have a naturally conceived child with a gene abnormality that no one knew about until the baby was born. Such parents may feel they are somehow devaluing their older child by deciding to use assisted conception to avoid the abnormality occurring again. Couples who have been advised their child has a 'suspect' gene, which has so far failed to manifest itself in a physical way, feel they are living with an unexploded but loudly ticking bomb just waiting to go off. Their inability to conceive a second child naturally then becomes both a loss and the reason they will avoid coping with this unexploded bomb.

Another situation that complicates grief about infertility is a couple's history of miscarriage or stillbirth. When treating IVF families, I have found the anxiety and grief much more difficult to treat when these very tangible pregnancy losses are added to the loss of natural conception. Many parents begin IVF treatment after multiple losses. Many have suffered repeated early miscarriages because embryos have failed to develop beyond the eighth or tenth week. Still others have reached a later stage in a pregnancy only to have a baby born far too early to survive. These parents often remain at the first stage of grieving, feeling numb throughout their losses, and are never able to move forward in their emotional coping. These feelings can seriously impact upon IVF success and, later, on parenting skills.

The third 'special' group of grieving couples are those who cannot conceive naturally and also cannot use IVF alone to conceive their child. These couples account for about 6 per cent of all those using IVF. Perhaps the woman fails to produce healthy eggs, her partner's sperm is of low quality or fertilisation is not successful. These are the couples, who, if they decide to try for an IVF child, must use a third-party donor, possibly a stranger.

When couples are desperate to conceive a child and have suffered through a long period of attempted natural conception, the prospect of receiving donor eggs, sperm or embryos may seem a straightforward choice between having a child and not having one. It seems a simple decision to make, and one that is often not explored too carefully for fear of failure. Sometimes it feels easier to ignore complex issues while focusing on achieving a most wanted goal. But once that goal is achieved and a healthy pregnancy results, couples report numerous feelings over the conception. How will the baby look and act and will he seem very different from his mother and father? How will they tell friends and family about the use of a donor? How will the parents cope when it comes time to explain his history to the child?

For all three 'special' groups of couples, professional counselling is important to help both partners explore what has happened to them, how they feel individually about the events surrounding infertility and how they deal with these feelings, both individually and as a couple. Grief reactions are often intense and unpredictable. Most couples lack the skills to resolve the complications alone. Without safe and gentle intervention, the issues fail to be discussed, each partner nurses his or her own hurts alone and a gulf forms between the couple.

Counsellors and psychologists with family and grief experience are most suitable for helping these special couples. Couples can approach their local mental health centre for information or ask for a recommendation from a friend or family member who has experienced a similar situation. Family doctors and hospital social work teams are also good sources for a referral to known and trusted professionals.

There are also sources of information and advice available on the internet. These sources are listed in the 'Useful Contacts' at the back of this book.

The couple relationship

Whatever the issues around the infertility, couples face intense stress that can derail the strongest of relationships. Most grieving couples are stressed and irritable and likely to strongly and sensitively react to any slightly negative comment that is made to them by well-meaning friends or family members. Furthermore, anger that is held deep down whilst a partner is at work or with people who do not know of the situation, may build up during the day so that the evening becomes a battleground as partners return home needing to vent these pent up emotions. A Canadian study into the experiences of 420 couples in 2006[3] along with other studies recently completed, clearly shows that men and women cope very differently with the trauma of infertility and that these differences can generate enormous frustration between partners at times. A man may become quiet and withdrawn or resort to searching the internet for answers whereas women often need to repeatedly talk through the situation needing to openly express grief.

Studies also show that stress makes partners feel more out of control, leading to greater conflict over issues that each partner can control. But this is not the way life has to be: there are a number of successful methods of reducing conflict and producing greater harmony despite the stress couples are undeniably facing.

Working on communication

Couples under stress rarely communicate effectively. They may believe they are saying what they feel clearly and listening carefully, but in practice emotions get in the way. A great deal of anguish can be avoided if partners take the time to think what they mean before beginning to speak and they ensure that the other has understood the true meaning of what has been said before reacting to the information.

As an exercise in renewing the strength of your relationship, practise better communication by giving each other a little time apart when you both return home. Then sit down somewhere quiet and spend ten minutes, with each of you in turn describing his or her day and how he or she is feeling. At the end of each turn, the listening partner relays what he or she has understood, to check that the meaning is clear to both. During this exercise, avoid blaming the other for miscommunication; instead, devise ways for both of you to improve. The more you practise this technique, the better your communication becomes and the less potential there will be for conflict.

Right or wrong

Another guaranteed fire-raiser is a partner telling the other how he or she should cope with feelings, or that these feelings should not exist at all. Every person will perceive loss in a slightly different way, will have feelings in different intensities and will experience relief from different strategies. The secret of a successful partnership is to navigate the stormy waters of infertility and its treatment together but in individual ways. It can be harder than it sounds.

Typical partner reactions to intense emotions are to 'make it better'. Men, particularly, like to 'do' something to jolly a partner out of the blues. This is rarely helpful and it may even make her angry. Similarly, telling a partner 'it's not that bad' when it clearly is communicates a lack of understanding that hurts.

A useful exercise in maintaining good boundaries in your relationship is to provide a listening ear while reminding yourself that it is your partner's responsibility to feel better when he or she is ready. I have had much success with simply focusing partners on providing physical comfort to meet distress rather than providing comprehensive solutions. Words may not help, and may even make things worse, when a hug alone communicates support and comfort without the likelihood of misunderstanding. And time spent watching a movie or a distracting television program cuddled together is often a wonderful treatment for distress.

Learn time out

Grief is intense and requires calm and time to ease. A grieving couple needs to ensure there is time in the day for quiet thought and simple pleasures. A gossip with friends over coffee, a walk in the country or by the beach, relaxing in bed with absorbing books to read or taking a long warm bath together are all good ways to nurture yourselves while allowing the grief to continue. Some grieving people are tempted to fill their lives with events or people in order to avoid thinking; this is rarely effective and can provoke intense anxiety. Even if you can only cope with being quiet and reflective for short periods, ensure this time is available.

Practise romance

A diagnosis of infertility seriously affects the quality of an intimate relationship. With partners feeling anything but attractive after being physically invaded and labelled, they could be forgiven for never wanting to have sex again. Even if neither partner feels that lovemaking is an option, keeping a romantic feel to your relationship is very important and extremely effective in strengthening coping skills.

Enjoying romance means expressing love and affection towards each other. Romance does not require huge planning or great monetary outlay. Romantic gestures are as simple as leaving a note in your partner's handbag saying 'I love you', buying the book he wanted and writing a message of affection inside or planning a candlelit dinner as a surprise. These gestures can help to overcome the damage to self-esteem most partners suffer with infertility.

Use others for support

Although a partner knows most about a loved one, he or she may not always be the best person to unload emotions on. As both partners are grieving in their own ways, one can easily become overwhelmed in trying to help the other. It is useful to maintain a mental list of close friends and family to talk to at the times when a partner seems overwhelmed, exhausted and unable to be supportive. Snapping or saying the other is unsympathetic will actually work in reverse, making the person feel more useless that ever.

Dealing with friends and family

A number of couples have reported that friends and family did not react to their plight as they would have wanted and that relationships were seriously strained at times or even ended. We always hope that those closest to us will be supportive and understanding allies during dark times, but the truth is that couples face many different responses to their infertility diagnosis and future treatment, some negative and some positive.

Many couples receive a great deal of advice from friends and relatives. This ranges from suggestions of different doctors to see and homeopathic remedies to try to the dismissive 'You'll be right, mate'. Although the advice will never totally cease, as this is very much human nature, there are ways to deal with it that make it less likely to be repeated. The most effective treatment for unwarranted advice is to calmly ignore it.

I am not suggesting that you flip your nose up at a friend, turn on your heel and run in the opposite direction. Rather, if you can simply move the conversation on to another, safer, topic so much the better. Alternatively, you can simply say, 'Thanks, that's interesting' and again rapidly change the subject. The worst technique to use with unwarranted advisors is to react with intense emotions because this increases the chance the advisors will repeat their mistakes.

A difficulty with family is that they may be too close to you, which means they are unable to be much support. One female patient of mine was faced with her mother who, every time she saw her, would burst into tears. This mother was so absorbed in her own grief she was completely unable to consider her daughter's needs. If family members and friends are seriously affected by your diagnosis, it is often wise to keep contact fairly superficial for a little while. Make visits a little longer as feelings begin to subside over time.

Several couples report they found family get-togethers a strain and at times even distressing. One couple had to attend a christening early on in their grieving process and found it 'just the longest day ever'. Families may have expectations that you are simply not able to fulfil. At times, the best way to deal with it can be to have a quiet chat with the hosts, explain that feelings are running high and ask that a more intimate celebration may be held a little later, aside from the main day. There may be a little tension over a non-attendance but having grieving prospective parents trying to cope on a day that is too emotionally demanding for them can be distressing for all concerned.

Another difficulty couples experience is the lack of knowledge their close friends have about how to help. This lack of understanding can lead to an avoidance of the grieving couple altogether, leaving them feeling even more isolated. Friends, especially those who are pregnant or have children, may feel unable to cope with the grief of infertility and may need reassurance from the couple themselves that their company is indeed helpful. Couples may also find it helpful to suggest to friends that they can be of assistance. Perhaps friends can provide an evening's distraction by coming to a movie or a weekend treat with dinner at a nice restaurant.

Many of the mothers I work with tell me that they are often scared to go near their friends at first for fear of breaking down in tears and 'making a fool of themselves'. As emotions can rise up quickly and sometimes without warning early in the grief process, they avoid personal contact to save the friend becoming distressed. In the end, this loss of support is detrimental to the healing process. It can be helpful to begin by seeing very close friends, explaining in advance that these are emotional days. That way, they will not be too surprised if you do become upset. Also reassure friends that they mean a great deal to you. As you become a little stronger, seek out other friends who may not have been able to cope with your emotions early on.

Religious and cultural pressures

Couples struggling with the issue of infertility and possible treatment options come from many backgrounds and religions. They often not only face pressures from family and friends but also from religious leaders and cultural norms. Many religions have a lot to say about various forms of assisted reproduction, and some hold unfavourable views of humankind's ability to manipulate nature.

The Catholic religion, for instance, has long viewed attempts to achieve conception in any way other than through intercourse of husband and wife as being against its basic principles. In 1987, the Vatican issued a statement about IVF, saying it was not acceptable, even though the Church accepts the use of fertility drugs. Protestants and Muslims often recognise artificial reproductive techniques, but only those using sperm and eggs from the married couple. Donor fertilisation is usually considered unacceptable. Jewish writers have adopted more liberal views, viewing any attempt to maintain fertility as a positive act.

There are more adverse views about embryos being frozen for later treatments. A number of religions do not entertain this process and view the disposal of unwanted embryos in the same manner as abortion. Other religions insist that the couple ultimately uses all embryos that result from an IVF treatment cycle in attempting to achieve conception.

Religious confusion is exacerbated by cultural norms. Some cultures and countries, such as Italy, have very strict regulations about IVF. Their near neighbours Spain and Egypt are much more relaxed. All these societal attitudes influence couples facing infertility and the options they have to overcome. Ultimately, the decision must be that of the couple alone.

Improving self-esteem

One of the most debilitating and longer term effects of infertility on couples is the blow this deals to self-esteem. Many studies have linked infertility to diminished feelings of self-worth, which do not improve without some effort on the part of both partners within the relationship.

Self-esteem is a measure of how we see ourselves in the world: our character strengths, our ability to form relationships, our practical and academic skills and our perception of how we appear to others. Self-esteem measures do differ between men and women due to different physical characteristics, brain processes and social norms. Self-esteem also stems from your upbringing: this is another difference when partners come from families with different values and cultures.

The American Psychological Association reports success using a psychological technique known as cognitive behavioural therapy (CBT) when working with women suffering lowered self-esteem due to infertility. This therapy relies on the fact that your thoughts very much influence your emotions, and that by helping to change your patterns of thinking your emotions will closely follow.

Women diagnosed with infertility receive negative messages about themselves, both actually and implied. There are increasing societal expectations of women managing to have careers, happy relationships and motherhood, at the same time and apparently all with ease. Women grasp these messages, thinking that because they are struggling with fertility, they are 'defective', 'stupid', 'physically less feminine' and somehow to blame. These thoughts lead to emotions of sadness, guilt and shame. CBT seeks to address these thoughts and turn the messages these women give themselves into more positive ones.

Most counsellors and psychologists are trained in CBT and may use it to help women through these issues by engendering a stronger sense of self-worth. Alternatively, women can try a few CBT exercises at home to determine if these ideas are of help to them.

CBT relies on writing down thoughts and feelings at regular times in the day, to help you become aware of your thought patterns and how the emotions follow. In practise, I have found busy women rarely have the time or energy to carry around a notebook wherever they go, scribbling furiously each hour on the hour. I have adapted the idea for busy women whose only time of peace is at night-time before they sleep. This is also a good time to write as it removes whirling negative thoughts from your mind, making them less likely to affect the quality of your sleep.

Buy yourself a journal, possibly a hardback notebook. Clients of mine have enjoyed making their journals personal by covering them in pretty paper. Make an entry each evening. First, mentally review the day: what you did and how you felt about yourself throughout this time. Next, focus on writing down the negative thoughts you had: what these thoughts were and what situations triggered them. Then write how the thoughts made you feel: perhaps a negative thought of 'I always feel alone even with people around' will make you feel sad and lonely.

Finally, beside each negative thought and emotion, write down a positive thought you would tell a close friend if she had said what you had thought. For example, if my best friend told me she always felt alone even when she was with a group of friends, I would tell her, 'You aren't alone. I'm really happy to talk to you and help you feel better supported.' Once I said this to her I guarantee she would feel less sad and less alone. This is the power of positive thinking.

Below is an example of journal entries:

Day	Negative thought	Emotion	Positive thought	Emotion
Monday, 23rd	'I'm alone even in a crowd.'	Sad, lonely	'A good friend will talk to me one-on-one.'	Less sad, more optimistic
Tuesday, 24th	'I messed up this report. I'm a failure.'	Worthless, not capable	'I will redo it now that I know what's required.'	Some feelings of achievement

'Positive-thought generation' takes practise before it is truly effective. Use it for several weeks before you decide whether it is right for you. The technique is one of the most powerful psychological tools we have and I find around four out of five women respond well to using it and that it significantly diminishes their anxiety and depression.

Most professions working with men who are dealing with infertility report that less is known about their feelings and how best to treat them for stress, anxiety and depression. It is often difficult for men to find a male psychologist who is experienced in fertility issues as few specialise in this field. However, I have successfully treated couples together for self-esteem issues arising from a diagnosis of infertility and I find this often works well.

If they cannot find a male psychologist, I implore men to try to meet another man who has also had infertility issues and get a talk going. Most men feel they are alone in not being able to father a child naturally, and this interferes with their masculinity and their ability to perform in the bedroom. Furthermore, invasive tests, although not as all-consuming as many women face, leave a man feeling 'not good enough'. Being able to share their feelings with someone who has faced a similar situation goes a long way to solving the stress.

It is also vitally important to ease the stress and raise self-esteem by re-negotiating lovemaking. Men who feel 'down-at-heel' after a battery of uncomfortable tests and negative results rarely feel sexy. Helping the couple see these feelings as normal, calling a temporary halt to full intercourse and instead exploring other ways of being intimate often restores *his* sense of worth and brings the partners closer together.

Men often say they feel they shouldn't have upsetting thoughts and feelings after a diagnosis of infertility, or even after a miscarriage. Resources for coping are predominantly aimed at women, and this causes men to feel they have no right to be 'not OK'. They also feel a need to stay strong to support their partner while forgoing their own needs. This is also detrimental to their self-worth and can be addressed simply by making men aware that, by having emotions, they are actually supporting and connecting with their partners and at the same time ensuring their own mental outlook is healthy.

Expressing distress and sadness is not solely a female trait, but an instinct designed to help us draw in support to survive and thrive. When couples talk about their feelings and accept each other's experiences of what they are going through, this will bring them together with added mutual respect. Respect from a partner also helps to raise self-esteem.

Controlling the uncontrollable

Coping with infertility also means learning ways to feel control in a situation where you feel you have none. Although I'm not advocating the use of a tight regime to contain the inevitable anxiety that arises with fertility issues, living with a pervasive sense of having no control is detrimental to mental health.

As we grow, we all develop a view of how we see the world and our role in it. We may feel that the world is predominantly uncontrollable by mere mortals and that we just have to accept what comes our way. Or we may live at the other end of the spectrum, believing that we completely control our destinies, and that if things go wrong it's because of our actions. Of course, it's rare to find people at such extreme ends of the scale: most of us feel that we have some control, although not over everything that happens. Where we fall on the scale is, however, very important in deciding how we might feel about fertility problems and what actions we take after a diagnosis.

The scale is an idea developed some fifty years ago by a psychologist called Julius Rotter. He called his idea the 'locus of control' and it is still well respected in psychological circles. The scale helps counsellors and psychologists identify how much people will 'bow to the inevitable' and do nothing or, alternatively, believe they can still alter outcomes.

If you believe strongly in fate, you have an external locus of control. A partner with a high external locus of control may well feel he or she is destined to be childless. This may lead to an examination of other options, such as a new and exciting career or expensive holidays and pets, to make up for the loss. On the other hand, a partner with a high internal locus of control will believe in leaving no stone unturned in his or her quest to achieve conception. Both extremes are apt to lead to anxiety and possibly later depression, as the situation is rarely black and white. In reality, couples suffering infertility do have some control in the form of informed choices to make, but they are rarely able to produce a desired result alone.

The best partnerships are those in which one partner favours a slightly internal pattern of control and the other tends towards the external. If positions are not extreme, partners then find it relatively easy to discuss their feelings and to establish a compromise. For example, the external partner may have left alone options of assisted conception if he were making the choice alone. However, his internal partner gives him renewed faith that a little more of their combined input will achieve a happy outcome.

Difficulties arise when one partner has a strong internal locus and the other a strong external locus of control. I have counselled couples when the internal partner is pushing in the direction of ever more tests and 'new' remedies to achieve natural conception. In the other corner, the external partner wants to accept the infertility and move to other options, such as IVF or adoption, or enjoying the child or children they already have. This can create much conflict, a great deal of hurt on both sides and an inability to form a compromise. In this instance, professional help is urgently needed to assist both partners to reflect on what has happened, how they feel and to evaluate all the available options in a responsible manner.

As a couple considering IVF treatment, reflecting on and talking about the infertility diagnosis or genetic problem, and what it means to each partner, can only empower you for the journey ahead. It is not at all about indulging in 'poor me'; rather, it is all about the mental preparation that will help you gain the most from IVF treatment.

2

Choosing IVF

One of the things I fantasised about during each cycle was getting 'fat'.

More than one million cycles of IVF begin every year throughout the world. The chance of success for each cycle is increasing and, currently, the overall average success rate of 21 per cent for all cycles rises to more than 35 per cent of all cycles for couples in their twenties and thirties.

Couples undergoing the process are not 'helpless'. There is evidence, both anecdotal and from large-scale research studies, to show there are many ways they can prepare to achieve success through IVF.

Healthy living

The first step for couples, after deciding that IVF might be the best option for their problem, is to improve the chances of a positive result by establishing a healthy lifestyle *before* treatment begins. Parents who worked on their health and fitness after a previous IVF failure report much better success the second time around. Not only will healthy living increase the chances of conceiving and carrying a baby to term, but it also helps couples cope with the psychological ups and downs of the process. As a prospective IVF couple, there are five steps for you to follow to achieve a healthy, balanced lifestyle.

Food for mind and body

Healthy eating does involve weight regulation: losing a few kilos if you are a little overweight or putting on weight if you are underweight can increase your chances of achieving conception, sometimes dramatically. Both partners should ideally have a body mass index (BMI) within the healthy ranges. BMI is calculated using both height and weight: it is easy to obtain a result using one of the many websites available. If your BMI is outside the healthy range, a visit to a dietician is an excellent starting point for advice on how to correct your weight. Losing weight is much easier with a supporting organisation such as Jenny Craig or Weight Watchers. If you feel you need more individual support, a counsellor can help you develop the psychological tools to effect lasting change.

Healthy eating is about getting the right foods. This means a variety of whole grains, fruit, vegetables, meat, dairy and a minimum of fatty foods each day. For a prospective mother, taking a folic acid supplement is extremely important to avoid neural defects and it has been shown to reduce the incidence of facial clefts by one-third. Also ensure you acquire enough iron: spinach once a week can help, as can meat eaten regularly. Adequate Vitamin C in the diet promotes iron absorption, so fruits such as oranges should be included. Iodine, important in preventing miscarriages, is found in dairy products and salt. Women preparing for pregnancy are advised not to drastically cut dairy and salt intake.

Healthy eating also means avoiding foods that may be implicated in diminishing fertility. An American study carried out for the Harvard School of Public Health demonstrates a link between infertility and the consumption of unhealthy fats (trans fats, which are found mostly in processed foods).[1] The aim is to eat fresh, unprocessed food, preferably organic.

Healthy eating can also protect your brain against stress. The brain contains chemical substances that help in stabilising your moods, minimising anxiety and depression. Stress can deplete these stabilising resources and eating a 'brain-healthy' diet can help to ensure the chemicals remain balanced. A diet rich in a substance called tryptophan is important because it crosses the barrier from the blood into the brain and is converted into the important brain chemical serotonin. Tryptophan-rich foods include dairy products such as milk, yoghurt and cheese, particularly Cheddar; meat, especially turkey; eggs; beans; fish, and oats.

Avoid or cut down on foods that contain substances with an anxiety-provoking or depressive effect on the brain, such as coffee and some carbonated drinks that contain caffeine, alcohol and highly sweetened foods. Caffeine has not been shown to adversely affect unborn babies if it is consumed in small quantities.

Stillness

Stress often makes us want to get busy to avoid confronting whatever is worrying us. However, busyness can make the worry significantly worse. Finding a time to be still every day can make stress much more bearable. Research has shown that taking time to reflect and deal with stressful experiences is an effective way to put them behind you.

Couples I have worked with have found many ingenious ways to be still: taking up yoga and meditation, keeping a daily journal, listening to a Mozart quartet, enjoying a quiet read, walking close to nature, gardening or relaxing in a bath each evening.

Healthy habits

Studies have shown that cigarette smoking seriously affects blood supply to the reproductive organs, making conception and maintaining a pregnancy much more difficult. Research has also proven that female smokers have poorer quality pre-ovulatory follicles, making it less likely that follicle stimulation, egg retrieval and attempted fertilisation will work. In fact, research suggests smoking adds ten years to a woman's reproductive age.

Choosing to stop smoking before trying for a baby using IVF will also be valuable for the health and well-being of your baby as he grows. Smoking can also increase anxiety, a fact that is very important to consider with IVF. If you are having difficulties quitting, get some professional support, such as contacting a helpline: trying to stop smoking on your own is often unsuccessful.

Exercise

Regular exercise keeps weight down, assists circulation and helps to prevent disease. Recent studies show good exercise habits before pregnancy can lessen the incidence of gestational diabetes, a problem that affects up to 10 per cent of mothers-to-be. On a psychological level, exercise is a very important antidote to anxiety and depression, boosting levels of natural painkillers and the 'feel-good' hormones known as endorphins. Exercise also reduces the levels of stress hormones circulating through the body. Adopting an enjoyable exercise routine can have enormous benefits to both partners undergoing IVF.

Passion

Passion is an intense emotion and one that compels action. Passion is a great energy-creator and it is of great benefit to anyone in a stressful period in life, particularly one that seems to overtake ordinary life completely. As you prepare for the challenges of IVF, get involved in something that takes you out of yourself, something you can be passionate about — perhaps rediscovering a musical skill or a sporting activity, going to the theatre or becoming involved with a craft — and use it as a diversion from everyday stresses and as a means of re-igniting your emotional life.

The right time

Couples say that finding the 'right time' to undergo IVF is not at all easy. Most feel they want to be free from everyday burdens. Prospective mothers, especially, feel an intense need to focus all their efforts on achieving a pregnancy and feel highly frustrated that normal events get in the way. And get in the way they do. It is worth both partners taking the time to talk through the coming eighteen months and agree a time that would allow both to mentally as well as physically prepare for the IVF process.

Horror times to avoid definitely include planned or existing house renovations, moving home, short-term caring for a sick relative, starting a new job and the first year after having a baby (conceived or adopted). These times are simply too disruptive to enable couples to focus on and cope with the stress of IVF.

Other considerations may include the time of year, particularly if one partner suffers seasonal affective disorder (in which a lack of sun and warmth brings on feelings of depression). Other times to avoid are the lead up to Christmas, which can be a most stressful time of the year, as well as sad anniversaries such as the death of a close relative or friend.

Deciding the right time also means taking the pregnancy into account, if a positive result occurs. When is the best time, particularly since nausea and tiredness may be problems? When would be a good time for the birth, what are the times that support people in your life may be most available to help and how does taking time off work to be with a new baby fit into long-term plans?

Many women preparing for IVF are using the technique because age has diminished fertility. Women aged thirty-eight and over are more anxious about the timing of IVF treatment, because they feel a heightened sense of urgency to achieve a pregnancy while they can. This urgency can seem overwhelming at times. I have talked to couples so focused on the need to begin treatment immediately that they were quite unable to focus on finding a time that was actually suitable. Urgency is normal and desired, but it is only useful to a certain degree. Success also depends on emotional and physical preparation and this may mean the couple take a few months to begin taking folic acid supplements, cease smoking and drinking alcohol, achieve healthy weights and identify sources of support.

If partners are finding it hard to cope with the preparation time, make a schedule of all the activities that will happen right up to implantation stage (see pages 46–47, 51–53). Begin work on fitness levels, develop a healthy eating plan and find time to be quiet. Have a program to follow on the wall or fridge and tick off each item as it is addressed. This organisation will help reduce the anxiety over fading fertility.

Financial considerations are also important in making a decision regarding the timing of IVF. You need to calculate all the costs of the treatment, for each cycle required, that are not funded publicly, as well as the normal costs of a pregnancy and of a healthy baby. Financial outlay can be considerable if several IVF attempts are required. Make sure the IVF clinic provides you with details of the full costs of treatment per cycle and check to ensure you are eligible to receive benefits. Before booking treatment, you need to know what costs are involved and when, so that you can plan ahead — and avoid sleepless nights and excessive stress.

The right place

Most countries require that IVF clinics be accredited with the assisted conception regulatory body. There are a number of internet sites that list accredited clinics in the top IVF-using countries such as the UK and US.

These sites are listed in the 'Useful Contacts' section at the back of this book.

When choosing a clinic, there are a number of issues to consider:

- A location fairly near to home will avoid long, stressful journeys when treatment is at its most intense.

- A facility that feels comfortable, with medical practitioners who are warm and reassuring, can make the whole process run much more smoothly. It is also very comforting to have a doctor who will happily answer questions and does not make patients feel they are delaying his or her time.

- A clinic with good success rates cuts down on the anxiety inherent in treatment. Couples can ask to see clinics' figures and use them for comparisons.

- Costs of treatment. Prices tend to be very similar from one clinic to another, but always ask to see a detailed description of fees for all the procedures that may be required and compare these with at least one other clinic.

- It is helpful if the clinic offers on-site counselling services. At times couples may feel quite distressed about the methods of treatment and a counsellor on the premises who can liaise with medical staff can be of great benefit.

It is a good idea to visit several clinics, talk to the doctors and get a feel for the different approaches to treatment and to the couples' well-being. Visiting several clinics can also provide a greater sense of peace with a chosen clinic once the decision is made. If partners disagree over a choice, it can be useful to talk over the issue with a third person, perhaps a friend or relative, to gain some perspective. Alternatively, making a list of the pros and cons of each clinic often identifies one as being better than the others.

Ask for support

Once both partners are happy with one clinic and a date that seems to be the best option in the circumstances, begin planning for the help needed during the treatment process. The process is less stressful if you have good support from friends and family and feel comfortable about asking for their assistance. You may need someone to go to each appointment with you or simply to drive you there, particularly if a partner cannot attend: people have expressed immense relief at having an ally for the egg and sperm retrieval and implantation phases (see pages 46–47, 51–53), which cause the greatest anxiety. Having some extra help around the house during the various phases of treatment is invaluable, particularly for the woman, who may be feeling low during the follicle stimulation phase and after implantation, when she would like to rest and give the pregnancy the best chance of success.

Many couples report feelings of intense isolation at times, even if there are other people around, and they get a great deal of comfort from talking to others experiencing IVF treatment. Women, particularly, feel different and are often left with the feeling that no one understands or cares. For help, enquire whether a chosen clinic has a support group operating. If the clinic has no group, consider starting one and asking clinic staff to publicise the idea. Alternatively, there are internet sites that allow couples to chat with others who are using IVF.

Telling the kids

Some couples planning IVF treatment may already have a naturally conceived child, an IVF baby or an adopted child. In blended families, one partner may have children from an earlier relationship. Many parents worry about the effect their treatment will have on their other child or children but lack the skills to prepare them in the best way.

A couple's first instincts may be to protect children by not telling them about IVF, especially if they fear failure. But this is rarely a successful strategy and can be harmful to the parent-child relationship. Children of all ages are very sensitive to their parents' emotions and will immediately sense unusual stress. They will then often assume the worst: a scenario far more frightening than IVF, such as a life-threatening illness, impending marriage break-up or the parent not loving them anymore.

If you are approaching IVF treatment and you have a child, you need to consider the child's age and stage of development before deciding how to approach the issue. The best guide to talking with children about adult topics is to give a little information and then see what happens. Perhaps explain that some parents, including you, need assistance from doctors to have a new baby. Watch your child to see how he uses the information, and tell him he can ask any questions he likes. Explaining basic facts of life to a young child may be helpful. For example: 'Mum and Dad want a baby, the doctor will help them and the baby will grow in Mum's tummy until he or she is big enough to come out.' To ensure the child feels part of the process, you could add, 'You have the important job of being big brother so the baby can learn things from you.'

Older children will want to know more and they often respond with lots of questions. It is helpful for parents to discuss likely questions with each other so they know how to answer and avoid awkward silences. Again, begin with simple ideas. Help your child to understand that some parents need help from doctors to make babies and that this is now common and routine. You do not need to describe the actual procedures, which may cause alarm, but be honest about where you are going when you keep appointments and describe what is happening in very basic terms. Children are adept at assimilating new information and are often less fazed by such processes than the adults around them. However, if your child seems particularly stressed or is engaging in attention-seeking behaviour during your treatment, it is worth employing some basic stress management tools for children. A great source of such ideas is Marti Belknap's book, *Stress Relief for Kids: Taming Your Dragons.*

Occasionally, parents are so traumatised or embarrassed by infertility and IVF they are unable to cope with talking to their children. Since trauma is easily passed on from parent to child, these parents should seek counselling before starting treatment to help them learn to cope with their own feelings and distress before they brief their children. Parents can contact their IVF clinic for advice or they may talk over their concerns with a private infertility counsellor.

Natural health

Although IVF is very much a medically based treatment process, natural therapies do have a very useful role for some couples, and should be considered and discussed with the IVF doctor before treatment begins. Some therapies may have adverse effects and it is essential to discuss their suitability with the clinic staff.

The most valuable contribution that natural therapies appear to make to the IVF process is the lessening of anxiety, depression and feelings of fatalism that can get in the way of the medical process. Researcher Daniel Campagne, in a paper published in the journal *Human Reproduction*, concludes, 'There is substantial initial evidence that the psychological disposition of the parents-to-be influences their fertility.'[2] Stress can affect a woman's fertility and decrease the quality of semen that men produce. Maintaining a healthy outlook on life is therefore of prime importance to couples undergoing IVF. Several therapies have been researched in conjunction with IVF in large reputable studies.

Acupuncture

Recent research has suggested that acupuncture promises improved success rates for couples going through IVF. Studies in both Denmark and Australia have shown that treatment can double the rate of IVF success. A growing number of enlightened clinics in the US have incorporated this therapy into their IVF treatment programs, and it is likely that other countries will follow suit. Further research is needed to determine exactly when during each cycle acupuncture is most effective. For further information about using acupuncture, discuss this option with your chosen IVF clinic. Staff may also be able to supply the name of a suitable practitioner.

Hypnotherapy

An Israeli study published in 2006 found hypnotherapy may double the chances of success with IVF.[4] However, the study had some limitations and so should not be taken as conclusive evidence that the effects of hypnotherapy are that significant. That said, hypnotherapy is employed in IVF programs in some British clinics and it is claimed it lowers levels of stress hormones, which can in turn increase pregnancy success. Hypnotherapy can also teach life-long relaxation skills that can improve your mood and maintain lower stress levels, especially during the years of trying to conceive and raising a young child. As with all therapies, find a practitioner who has a recognised qualification and experience in treating couples going through IVF.

Counselling and stress management

Stress hormone levels, particularly of the female partner, are greatest around the collection and implantation periods (see pages 46–47, 51–53). An experienced IVF counsellor, Kay Oke, reports that women undergoing treatment have similar stress levels to those coping with a life-threatening illness. 'Stress levels during IVF treatment can become obstacles to effective living,' she says. Stress management techniques and effective counselling can decrease effects of stress and create a more stable life for both partners.

All couples should have counselling during the IVF process. The two main reasons are to maintain the integrity of the couple's relationship and to reduce feelings of fatalism and negativity that almost always occur. Instability in the relationship and negativity are major causes of couples dropping out of IVF programs and also have serious long-term effects on the ability to parent happily and successfully.

Counselling and stress management should be tailored to meet the needs of the individuals concerned, but all care plans have six basic items.

- *Keeping a journal:* I encourage both partners to keep a journal, perhaps writing two or three sentences detailing their thoughts and emotions at the end of each day (see page 23). Recording thoughts and feelings is a good way of calming your whirling thought patterns, improving concentration and promoting restful sleep.
- *Identifying close supports:* Couples rarely think about other people they can turn to when their partner is not available or unwilling to provide support. The stresses of everyday life, work and IVF treatment can make someone physically or emotionally 'unavailable'. Rather than feeling resentment, the person needing comfort or a listening ear should turn to someone they trust until their partner is 'available' again. One person can never meet another's needs all the time, no matter how easy or difficult life is. The counsellor will help each partner assess who is the best kind of support at times of intense emotion, investigate people who may be suitable, and help partners decrease the anger they may feel when a partner cannot support them all the time.

- *Identifying useful coping strategies from past events*: One psychological technique that is very helpful in dealing with IVF stress is for both partners to focus on other occasions in life when they have been stressed, the methods they used to cope then and how successful they were. Typically, people report being stressed over exams, when they first left home, over the break-up of relationships and during separations from a partner. Ideas that have been proven to work can be successfully employed in the IVF treatment process.

- *Learning to express feelings*: By the time couples arrive at the beginning of IVF treatment, they have already been through an emotional time. Along the way, each has found different coping styles, which at times have generated anger with each other because their views differ. The result of this anger is to reduce the amount and quality of communication within the relationship. In the counselling environment, couples can explore what is happening to them, their individual feelings and any misperceptions they hold about how the other is coping. At times of stress, it is easy to interpret a partner's anger at the invasiveness of treatment or the loss of a pregnancy as anger directed towards you.

- *Learning deep breathing technique*: One of the fastest and most effective ways to reduce levels of stress is to alter your breathing patterns. When stressed, humans tend to breathe faster and more shallowly. Becoming aware of these patterns and changing them in response to stress is a very useful technique. If you are feeling anxious during the IVF treatment, take time out to lie down comfortably on your back with your head on a pillow. You can be on a bed, sofa or floor — but make sure you are comfortable. Place a hardback book on your stomach. Now take a deep breath in for six seconds, deep enough to make the book rise. Exhale also for six seconds, allowing the book to fall. Repeat for ten minutes. Notice how you feel in this more relaxed state. Practise regularly and you will eventually be able to deep-breathe standing up, at work, in the bus queue or in a meeting.

- *Learning conflict resolution*: Stress raises the nervous system into a more 'excited' state, where it is much easier for tempers to be frayed. Once couples become aware that conflict is almost inevitable when they are stressed, they can learn methods of diffusing this inevitable anger. There are three useful 'rules' to minimise conflict. In an argument, avoid bringing in past events and hurts; instead, stick to the present. Avoid criticising a partner: if you find behaviour upsetting, say, for example, 'I feel hurt when you are late home and you don't call me. Could we talk about ways we can keep in touch more regularly?' This avoids the disagreement spiralling out of control. And learn to take time out when anger rises: it is wise to tell a partner when feelings are spiralling out of control, ask for a little space and set a later time for the discussion. Then take a walk or practise deep breathing until control is restored.

3

The Stages of IVF

I was very aware of my body and I needed to rest a lot.

Before treatment begins, it is important to have written details of the procedures each partner will undergo so that both can anticipate what is coming and are able to plan accordingly. The IVF clinic should provide this to all couples who are undergoing treatment. Although, at the time of an appointment, verbal instructions may seem fine, many people report feeling forgetful and unsure as the process continues. Also bear in mind that the process is stressful, and stress can easily make partners doubt their own recollections of what has been said.

Although every IVF treatment is tailored to meet the special needs of an individual couple, there are a number of procedures each couple will likely undergo:

- A counselling session is mandatory for couples living in some jurisdictions.
- Stimulation of the ovaries to produce eggs, using hormones administered orally, by nasal spray or by daily injection. This stage is not used for

couples using frozen embryos, natural fertility cycles or the newer in vitro maturation (IVM).

- Daily blood tests and several pelvic ultrasound examinations.
- Administration of an egg-ripening injection if stimulation is used.
- Egg collection one to two days later, usually under a light general anaesthetic if a stimulated cycle is being used.
- A sperm sample from the male, usually at the same time as the egg retrieval for stimulated cycles. If problems have occurred with the production of sperm, such as a blocked vas deferens, sperm can be collected via a medical procedure.
- The combination of the sperm and eggs to allow fertilisation to take place. A single sperm may be injected into the egg to increase the chance of fertilisation, a technique known as intracytoplasmic sperm injection (ICSI).
- Embryos that do develop tested for abnormality.
- One or two embryos implanted in the female's womb. Other viable embryos may be frozen.
- Hormone therapy given to the woman to maintain the best environment for pregnancy to occur and endure.

Each of these stages involves particular stresses.

Most couples report finding the stimulation phase emotionally tiring. The female partner can feel anxious about what is happening to her body. One woman reported, 'My body was already working overtime because of the various drugs and was nearly becoming over-stimulated.'

Many women report being worried that the hormones will not work and that the high concentrations may do harm either to their bodies or to the embryoes once they are implanted. There is no conclusive evidence that the treatment poses long-term risk, but anecdotal evidence suggests there may be an increased risk of cancer for some women who have undergone

IVF, prompting advice that regular breast examinations and PAP smears are undertaken.

The stimulation stage of treatment is changing with new technology. Recent research suggests that high doses of stimulating drugs may not increase the chances of achieving suitable eggs (compared with lower doses) and may even pose the risk of over-stimulation. Furthermore, British studies suggest that very high stimulation of the ovaries may reduce the quality of the eggs harvested. Some couples are able to use a natural female cycle without drugs to collect an egg, a process that can also diminish the cost of treatment. Two recent studies of IVF pregnancies showed that couples using a natural female cycle or very low stimulation cycle for egg collection were just as likely to conceive as those who were using stimulating drugs.[1] Couples expressed a much greater preference for the natural cycle over stimulation when this was feasible.[2] Research has suggested that another benefit to be gained from using a natural cycle is a healthier birthweight for babies compared with weights after stimulation cycles.

Another new and potentially beneficial technique to avoid the use of the egg stimulation phase of treatment is called in vitro maturation (IVM). Researchers have found a method of taking immature eggs from a woman, ripening them in a culture in the laboratory and allowing fertilisation to take place when sperm are introduced. Studies of the IVM procedure suggest that success rates are not significantly different from those achieved through IVF.[3] However, this method may result in higher pregnancy rates for women with polycystic ovary syndrome, who often cannot use ovarian stimulation, and it may also reduce the cost of treatment for suitable couples.

If the woman does require stimulating drugs, she may feel particularly stressed. The drugs given and the need to have painful injections daily can result in emotional highs and lows.

Egg retrieval and sperm donation bring new challenges, but can also mark a positive phase in which both partners feel they are progressing towards their goal. 'I felt I was finally getting somewhere,' one woman said of the news that four eggs had been successfully collected. 'The difficulties of the earlier weeks seemed very much worthwhile,' she said. At this point, the male partner becomes involved, producing a sperm sample, and this can lessen possible resentment building up in the initial phase where a female feels she is 'doing all the work'.

The time waiting to discover if fertilisation has taken place, and if there are viable embryos to use, is one of the most difficult periods of treatment. Uncertainty is the hardest situation to deal with and most couples report life very much 'standing still' over this time. They also report having poor concentration and little interest in life outside of the IVF clinic. Surviving this time with emotions intact requires a mix of healthy distraction by friends, work and gentle exercise, together with time spent talking about emotions. Using the relaxation skills outlined above (see pages 40–42) can also assist during waiting.

Typically, feelings become positive if embryos do develop. Studies have shown that couples with embryos to implant, possibly with 'spares' to freeze for later attempts, have the most positive outlook on life of all couples using IVF.[4]

How many?

Before 2005, one in four cycles of IVF treatment produced twin or triplet babies, most of whom were born prematurely. This was due to the common plan of implanting two or more embryos per cycle in the hope of increasing the chance of success. The increased resources needed to care for premature multiple babies added to the increased risk posed to a mother going through a multiple pregnancy has led to widespread legislation limiting the number of embryos implanted in each cycle. Many IVF authorities, such as the UK's Human Fertilisation and Embryology Authority, limit implantation to one embryo per cycle. Other authorities have guidelines about the number of embryos transferred that clinics adhere to.

Although many couples have confided to me that they wished they were able to transfer more than one embryo each cycle, the consequences of a twin pregnancy can be devastating. After losing one of her babies, a mother of twins reported, 'The IVF clinic had recommended that we only transfer one embryo so I felt it was my fault for asking for two.' Such tragedies affect families deeply.

Couples are often reassured by the evidence of recent studies that show transferring more than one embryo per cycle is unlikely to increase the odds of success. The technological advances made in the screening and selection of embryos and the better conditions in which embryos are kept before transfer has ensured that pregnancy rates are greater than ever before. This is especially true for women aged thirty-five and under who use IVF. Some countries do allow two embryo transfers in exceptional circumstances such as for a much older mother.

Genetic investigations

The number of embryos available for implantation or freezing may be reduced but of a higher quality if the couple elects to undergo pre-implantation genetic diagnosis (PGD). In this process, carried out after fertilisation, one or two cells are removed from the developing embryo for analysis. Generally, the cells can be checked for genetic abnormalities within twenty-four hours of the sample being taken. PGD is recommended for couples who know they have, or are carriers of, a genetic disorder that could prove harmful to a baby. PGD may also be suitable for those who have experienced unexplained miscarriages or multiple unsuccessful IVF attempts. It is thought that choosing embryos with no evident abnormality will significantly improve the chances of success.

There is little observed risk from this testing procedure, although waiting for PGD results is an additional period of uncertainty. However, this can be more than offset by the knowledge that the implanted embryo or embryos will not carry a genetic problem, which will reduce anxiety during a pregnancy.

Advanced testing of eggs, sperm and embryos are likely to become routine procedures in IVF clinics in the future. Improvements are being adopted every year: for example, recently new technology facilitating more detailed examination of egg structures has been trialled. The ability to detect optimal eggs, sperm or embryos will significantly increase the chance of a successful pregnancy.

Some parents have reported guilt and grief associated with embryos or eggs that were found to have abnormalities and could not be implanted.

Donation

For 6 per cent of the couples who undergo IVF, reproduction is vastly complicated by the need to involve a third party in the treatment process. The issues involved in using donor eggs, sperm or embryos are complex. Many couples have successfully used donation to achieve a family and have adored the baby who arrived. However, being alert to the feelings they may face, together with strategies to manage these feelings and avoid conflict, will ease the difficulties the couple may experience.

American psychologist Linda Applegarth, an expert on donor issues, believes that taking the time to come to terms with the need for donation will assist families to become comfortable with their decision.[5] She emphasises that couples may need to wait up to six months after learning that donation is necessary before being ready to face the challenge of fertility treatment. Emotional reactions to the need for a donor often include anger and despair at the failure to conceive naturally, grief that the expected child will not arrive and heightened fears about bonding with the child waiting to be born.

Prospective parents may not be able to resolve all these issues before conceiving but, by acknowledging the complexities and trying to establish how they do feel about donation, they may lessen their impact. Some fears about conception, pregnancy and birth through donation are inevitable. Many worry that the relationship with their child may not develop normally. In my experience, this only happens if parental feelings are 'locked away' and not expressed. Before attempting to conceive, it is worth reading Caroline Lorbach's book *Experiences of Donor Conception Parents, Offspring and Donors Through the Years*, which covers all of the issues raised by those involved with donation and provides guidance on what parents can expect, from before IVF right through the years of parenting.

Many couples using donors spend time on a waiting list before receiving the eggs, sperm or embryos they need to undergo IVF treatment. This can be a frustrating and lonely time. Women tend to have stronger emotional reactions during the waiting period than men do, but both partners may feel better if these emotions are allowed full expression, even though nothing can be done to change the wait. Trying to hold emotions in and to put on a 'brave face' is not sound preparation for a pregnancy.

This forced waiting time is a good opportunity to prepare yourselves carefully for the treatment: eating wisely, establishing a regular exercise routine, taking time out to be together and enjoying social time with friends. This is also a good time to seek counselling with a trained infertility counsellor.

Generally, donors are matched with blood type and some physical traits. Parents may feel anxious about the characteristics their child will have and may have some choices in the matter. There are two sides to the nature versus nurture debate, but there is little doubt that a child raised with love and wisdom will flourish.

Embryo preservation

Most couples who have spare embryos from the initial stimulation cycle of IVF will want to have these preserved for later attempts, or for another child if pregnancy does occur with the first cycle. Preservation removes the need for the woman to go through the follicle stimulation and egg retrieval processes again

The usual method is to freeze the embryos in specific solutions over a period of several hours to avoid cell damage. Generally, a single embryo is frozen in a separate vial for ease of use after thawing. Prior to freezing, embryos are graded to ensure that the most viable can be identified. New techniques, which may reduce the impact of freezing on embryo quality and increase the likelihood of thawed embryos being implanted success-fully, are under development. They include a 'snap-freeze' technique known as vitrification, which appears to be of greatest benefit for older women.

Embryo preservation often evokes unease, which many people choose to avoid. They may wonder whether the freezing process affects the baby that might eventually be born, or what changes occur to the embryo when freezing happens, but they rarely articulate such feelings. Parents have difficulty knowing how to think about the frozen embryos: as part of themselves, as separate living beings or as potential life existing in suspended animation.

Women generally appear to be more ready to deal with these complexi-ties than men do. Perhaps part of the reason for this is because it is the woman who will have the thawed embryo implanted in her womb if the couple require this. This physical closeness of the embryo may focus her thoughts on what has occurred to it previously. These issues may be more difficult for the man because, to him, the embryo appears to be much less tangible.

If, during the IVF process, you have concerns about freezing spare embryos, raise the issue with your clinic counsellor. Some couples, perhaps for religious reasons or other personal beliefs, cannot cope with the concept and should explore other options if they want children. However, the frozen embryo decision is straightforward if both partners agree. When couples have conflicting views over such delicate issues, emotions can run extremely high.

Embryos frozen for up to thirteen years have been thawed and successfully implanted. There are several options for embryos no longer needed: disposing of them, donating them to couples who cannot produce embryos or donating them for scientific research. This issue is explored more thoroughly in Chapter Nine (page 171).

Implantation

Implantation of the embryo in the womb was traditionally attempted on the third day after fertilisation had taken place. However, new research suggests that an embryo transferred on day five (termed a blastocyst) is likely to be more successful. Transfer times may vary due to embryos developing differently.

Many parents-to-be are very positive about implantation day, feeling that at last they are on the way to becoming parents. 'I just wanted to nurture myself, to give that precious collection of cells every bit of energy I could,' said one woman, who had arranged for a friend to come over and make the couple dinner. Some fathers-to-be reported wanting to wrap their partners in cotton wool. Couples are usually told that normal activity and even sex is perfectly acceptable. However, it is recommended that a woman avoids getting very hot or performing exercises that leave her gasping for breath. She may feel the need to take a day or two off work so she can come to terms with the procedure.

Then comes the waiting: of around two weeks before a pregnancy blood test can be performed. All IVF couples talk about this period in hushed tones, recognising it is both exciting and terrifying. 'I found it so hard to get those little cells off my mind for the first few days,' one woman said. 'All day, every day, I would be trying to imagine what was going on in there and willing with all my strength for those embryos to be OK.'

Using the coping strategies you have learned earlier helps at this anxious time. It can also be helpful to listen to a relaxation tape each day, music or a meditation designed to achieve body and mind relaxation. Some people find such tapes more helpful than others, but any relaxation achieved is very worthwhile, both to assist in implantation and to reduce the longer term effects of stress on mind, body and relationships.

Many women are acutely sensitive to how their bodies feel during this waiting period. They review every feeling, trying to establish if they are sensing physical changes brought about by pregnancy. They may feel absolute elation one morning because their breasts feel particularly sensitive and desperate by dinner time because the feeling has vanished. It is wise to expect many mood changes during these two weeks due to your own sensitivity and the treatment process. Try to keep an open mind, note the feelings — perhaps write them in a journal — and view them as part of the process. And say this 'mantra' to yourself: 'I am going to allow any and all of my feelings to come and then to go. I will not hold on to a feeling until the day of my test. Until then I will relax and let my body be.'

The test

IVF clinics always advise clients not to use store-bought pregnancy tests because these can offer a false-positive reading due to the hormones used to assist implantation. It is very tempting to try to find out as early as you can if the treatment has been successful, but this can cause acute and unnecessary grief.

The blood test is generally taken in the morning and results obtained by the end of the day. Prepare for discovering the result: be together as a couple when you are informed or have a support person there with you.

Your reactions to the result — either way — will probably be extreme. The pressure has been building from the time you acknowledged infertility problems right through the course of the treatment. You have had to deal with many emotions. You may have a reaction very different from the one you expected to have. But there are no 'right' or 'wrong' ways to react.

A negative

Failure is only the opportunity to begin again more intelligently.

— Henry Ford

There is no doubt grief will be felt after a negative pregnancy test. You may experience anger, intense sadness, a feeling that the result is not real and be simply overwhelmed. Although these initial feelings can seem too strong to bear, time will make them feel just a little easier to cope with.

Gather support from people you feel comfortable with. You may want periods of quiet, or someone alongside who does not make any demands. Initially, do not expect much of yourself. Try to grieve fully, as that makes it easier to decide on a way forward later.

Avoid making plans immediately. Neither of you will feel ready to commit to a plan for a few weeks. Postpone discussions about what you wish to do next until the first intense pain has receded just a little. Care for yourself by trying to eat well, sleep well and exercise a little.

Research shows that, once the initial shock and pain has eased, people who can maintain a problem-solving approach fare better psychologically than people who become fatalistic.[6] To engage in problem-solving, first arrange a meeting with your doctor to talk through the treatment and any test results that may be relevant. Write down any different approaches that may be suggested so you and your partner can talk them over privately. Further tests may be helpful before attempting a further IVF cycle: there are possible immunological problems that can interfere with implantation, and these can be treated.

It is very important to understand that, typically, IVF treatment is not a one-cycle process. Although some couples do achieve a pregnancy with the first attempt, many more do not. Swedish research suggests that, realistically, couples should be prepared for up to three cycles to achieve a pregnancy.[7] The likelihood of successful conception after three cycles is estimated to be 65 per cent, much higher than the figure for a single cycle, which is around 35 per cent, depending on the woman's age.

If age is not a consideration, you may like to think about taking a break from treatment for a few months. Going on a holiday to change your surroundings, so you can relax and recover your intimacy with each other, can be helpful.

At this time, you may also be evaluating other options apart from IVF. Some couples are focused on trying IVF until they succeed, whereas others may feel they are ready to consider adoption or even surrogacy. Try to keep an open mind, evaluate all the choices and listen to each other's point of view even if you may not agree with it. If you do decide to try IVF again, review your choices, such as your satisfaction with the clinic and the timing, and consider other stressors in your life which may need managing. Also review ways to improve your physical and mental preparedness with exercise and natural therapies.

Allow your emotions to come and go during this period of reflection after the test result. Many couples, women especially, report feelings they experience as 'crazy', such as intense anger or even hatred for a relative who has suddenly become pregnant or another couple who has achieved a pregnancy through IVF. Such feelings are very normal in your situation and should be openly acknowledged and discussed. If you feel you cannot talk to your partner or family, consult your counsellor.

4

Being Pregnant

I was very nervous and did not want to see any doctors or have any tests or procedures until I felt the babies were past the 'danger' period.

Olivia simply did not believe it. She remembered the nurse talking to her on the telephone and nothing sinking in. 'She could have been talking in Swahili for all I knew,' Olivia said, reflecting on that day two years ago. 'I felt like it was happening to someone else. Later, the joy really took hold.'

Couples can always recount the day they discovered a much longed-for pregnancy. They will remember the place and time, even the smells and sensations they were taking in. 'I was deliriously happy, but it was also a life-changing event,' reported the mother of a twin boy and girl. 'Finding out' is a moment burned in the brain for eternity.

After the initial delight, numbness often follows. They may think they were dreaming, floating through space or even experiencing an out-of-body sensation. This is the brain's way of reducing the impact of shocking news. It is as if it wraps itself in cotton wool for a while, diminishing the power of information coming in and going out. This feeling may last hours or days, depending on the person and the amount of time, effort and pain that has gone into achieving the conception. It will end only when couples are ready to face the reality.

First-trimester anxiety

'During IVF, when the eggs were collected and as we waited to see if fertilisation would happen, I really visualised pregnancy as being this time when I'd sit around with my feet up, a contented smile on my face at what I'd achieved,' an IVF mother told me. 'It just wasn't like that. The minute the pregnancy sank in, I felt panic. Within a few weeks, a sense of loss followed. I no longer had the daily checks, blood tests and clinic nurses to talk to which had been a facet of life undergoing IVF for all three of our attempts across two-and-a-half years. Suddenly, I felt completely on my own.'

People who have never experienced IVF always expect that a successful pregnancy test after one or more treatment cycles will trigger joyous celebrations right up until the birth. After all, pregnancy is what was wanted. That does not happen with most couples I have worked with. Joy and celebration are definitely a feature of the first days after the pregnancy is confirmed. However, often this is quickly followed by bouts of overwhelming anxiety. It is anarchy in the mind: a thousand worries jump out of nowhere at odd moments. 'Desperate to keep this miracle baby and terrified that it isn't going to last,' was how one woman summed up her feelings in early pregnancy. Knowing what to expect and how to deal with these worries reduces the strain on body and mind and helps to make pregnancy a more positive experience.

Typically, the early weeks of pregnancy produce times of intense anxiety until after the crucial twelve-week milestone, when the risk of miscarriage is drastically reduced. Most couples want to keep the pregnancy private during this time.

Many women express the fear, whether IVF was used or not, that telling everyone before the twelve weeks will somehow jinx the pregnancy. A male partner needs to be sensitive to the woman's feelings about this and discuss any revelations he wants to make about the expected baby *before* they are made, even to family. Most couples find the best option is to tell a few close family members or friends so that there is support available for both partners.

For the woman, much of the early anxiety centres on her body and whether or not it is up to the task of carrying the baby to term. This is a very normal fear and one that is exacerbated for women who are anxious by nature and for those who have suffered a miscarriage previously. The anxiety may be normal but it needs to be addressed if the pregnancy is to have the best outcome. Studies have shown that maternal stress hormones do cross the placenta, entering the foetal bloodstream. It is now accepted that this anxiety can affect the baby, leading to a more sensitive newborn. There is also evidence that severe anxiety can lead to premature birth. Although this is not common, it is worthwhile investing the time to learn anxiety reduction techniques.

For a prospective father, an IVF pregnancy brings on the typical anxieties, namely, 'Will I be able to be a good father,' and 'Will I be able to provide for my child's future?' The assisted conception can make these anxieties worse, coupled as they are with the man's concern over what his partner's body has been through already during the IVF treatment and will go through in pregnancy and birth. Again, it is worth investing in anxiety reduction strategies to ensure that the male partner can support his mate effectively.

There are two main avenues to containing the anxiety over a new assisted pregnancy. The first is finding a safe pair of medical hands to care for mother and baby throughout the pregnancy and birth. The second is the introduction of a 'worry-less' lifestyle.

The medical practitioner

Once a pregnancy has been confirmed by the IVF clinic, care is generally handed over to the couple's chosen obstetrician who will look after the mother and baby and often be present at the delivery. Couples may also book into a public hospital for antenatal care and delivery.

Many IVF couples feel a sense of bewilderment over the move from the fertility clinic to obstetrician. 'This pregnancy had been so hard to achieve, it was so precious, we felt as though someone should be watching over us to make sure all was well the whole time,' reported an IVF couple shortly after receiving the good news. Many couples feel that their unique and often very arduous path to prospective parenthood should require more careful observation. Couples are well within their rights to ask their medical practitioner for this.

For most IVF parents, the choice of doctor is a hugely important one. After all, this is the first person a couple will turn to if there is a problem with the pregnancy. Couples report they need quick access to this doctor if there are concerns, and adequate time at each appointment to discuss all the worries that may surface.

If you have just discovered a pregnancy after IVF, it is well worth interviewing a few obstetricians before making a choice. Note how a doctor's receptionist deals with your enquiry when you call, find out the average waiting time for an appointment, discuss your specific needs with the obstetrician and ensure he or she understands you will have worries that can only be eased by medical checks. Ensure the doctor has a good bedside manner and takes the trouble to explain technical issues.

At the first appointment, discuss the frequency and nature of checks you will have throughout the pregnancy. Many IVF parents are reassured by slightly more frequent visits than are usual for normal pregnancies, plus an ultrasound if there are any problems such as spotting or bleeding. Also discuss additional tests that may be carried out, such as blood tests and amniocentesis.

If you cannot afford a private medical practitioner, discuss your need for reassurance and continuity of care with your chosen hospital. There is usually some scope within the public health sector for increasing the amount of checks that you have and also having a designated contact in case of concerns.

Lifestyle changes

Adopting a less worrisome life will benefit both partners — and ultimately unborn children too. Begin by trying out one or two of the ideas suggested, gradually building up more techniques as time passes.

- For the first twelve weeks, be highly conscious of *what you have to do and what you want to do*. While you are coming to terms with a positive result and awaiting the twelve-week mark, do only what has to be done. Leave the 'wants' written down on a list taped to the fridge for a quieter time in your life.
- *Eat for calm*. What you consume can have a significant effect on how worried or how calm you are. In times of greatest stress, it is always a good idea to reduce caffeine intake, as this is one of the biggest triggers for increased anxiety and losing sleep. Avoiding alcohol is advised with all pregnancies. Eat regular small meals throughout the day to maintain a stable blood sugar level. And drink plenty of water to maintain hydration.
- *Plan your life in advance*. Anxiety is made much worse by sudden changes in routine. Keep a calendar on the wall and ensure that you write down commitments well ahead of their scheduled time. Avoid too many close together, and instead plan for some time to be quiet each and every day.
- *Exercise to feel calm*. Research has shown exercise to be one of the best ways of reducing anxiety. A walk together each evening can work

wonders and this will also help to reduce early pregnancy symptoms such as nausea.

- *Engage in relaxing activities every day.* Sit down together and cuddle up while you mull over the events of the day or go out for a meal when you feel too tired and emotionally drained to prepare food. Watch a comedy on television, or immerse yourself in an absorbing book, which is especially beneficial for anyone experiencing difficulty sleeping.

The fear of loss

Couples may also experience fears of loss during the first trimester. These fears can be triggered by the woman experiencing pain or spotting or may occur at the stage at which a previous miscarriage occurred. All can induce a full-blown panic reaction in a prospective parent.

In this situation, information is crucial for the couple's well-being. There are many myths about pregnancy and as many so-called experts willing to tell them. Rather than believing everything you hear, ensure you have good information. For example, early bleeding is not uncommon in pregnancy and studies suggest it may be more likely with IVF. It does not always imply a problem. Seek medical advice before you begin imagining the worst and note there is no evidence that assisted conception adds to the risk of pregnancy loss. A male partner can be very helpful at this time, reminding his partner not to regard the situation as a catastrophe.

Visualise the positive: women who have experienced miscarriage are naturally nervous at the same time in a later pregnancy. Rather than feeling helpless, having a positive picture of your pregnancy will calm you. Picture your baby gently moving around inside you. Take slow, deep breaths and imagine yourself sending messages of support to your baby. Breathe and picture your baby smiling at your loving care. Repeat this visualisation twice a day and whenever you feel the anxiety rise.

Discovering envy and anger

The first trimester can also bring distressing feelings of unexpected envy and anger. Most IVF parents report feelings of envy at times as they meet other pregnant couples who have conceived naturally. 'I was very envious of other women who had become pregnant naturally and seemingly without effort or thought,' one IVF mother said. These feelings of envy are very normal in the circumstances. Often, simply expressing these feelings to each other, or to a confidante or to a counsellor, and having a valued person listen is enough to substantially reduce the impact of these feelings.

Most IVF parents also feel anger during the first trimester and are shocked at the presence of such an 'inappropriate' emotion. Yet anger is a very normal emotion and is often a way of masking fear. The fear can relate to many different feelings: that the pregnancy won't succeed or fear that it will, that parenthood will be terrible despite the time and effort invested to make it happen.

The way in which anger is handled can minimise its destructive power. To ensure anger is used wisely, it is sensible to avoid reacting to the emotion immediately. If you both experience anger during the pregnancy, take time out to explore the feeling. Write down your thoughts and decide how to gain strength from anger. Decide you will nurture yourself when you are fearful and talk to your partner about these fears. If anger does not dissipate, it may be wise to seek a few counselling sessions to work on the problems behind the anger.

It's not my baby

Special circumstances surrounding a conception may result in particular feelings that may complicate the pregnancy. One of the most difficult issues is that arising from a conception using donor eggs, sperm or embryos.

Many couples are very focused on achieving a healthy pregnancy and are rarely able to explore the ramifications of donor-aided conception until they are well into the second trimester. It is often around the time when the first flutters of movement are felt that both partners may experience complicated emotions.

Linda Applegarth, director of psychological services at the American Center for Reproductive Medicine and Infertility, reports that egg and sperm donation represents a loss to couples of a chance to have their own child, a loss that must be grieved as any other.[1] Once the pregnancy is well established, this loss may profoundly affect couples, provoking symptoms of sadness, anger and depression.

Partners will cope with this grief in different ways. The woman usually needs to talk her feelings over with those she trusts, she will need to cry and perhaps keep a diary, writing down her feelings as they come and go. For the father, his loss will be about missing the chance to pass on his DNA, and he may react with shock, denial and sometimes anger. He may experience intermittent sexual dysfunction because the loss affects his identity as a male. It is important for both partners to share their feelings but also recognise other supporters are needed to avoid overloading each other. Women can be helped by other women, and, in the same way, men can benefit from talking to male friends who may have struggled with infertility issues. Both partners need to understand they are not alone in the stressful experience they are negotiating.

If issues over donor-assisted conception do not ease over the second trimester, the couple will benefit from undergoing counselling together. Talking to each other about the feelings that accompany the traumatic loss of a biological child offers a positive chance of facing up to that loss. The counsellor will set tasks for both partners, designed to help each to grieve the loss in a healthy fashion and to enable the couple to look forward to the birth positively.

It won't be normal

Most pregnant women report fears over whether or not their babies will be normal. As the pregnancy progresses, many women suffer frightening dreams of handicap or malformation. But mothers who have been through IVF seem to suffer these dreams and feelings more than other women do.

After IVF treatment, parents often feel the process was unnatural. They fear that the techniques used to harvest the eggs, collect the sperm and prepare for fertilisation may have damaged the embryo. IVF mothers also fear that the drugs used to stimulate ovulation and ensure implantation of the embryo may also harm the unborn baby. If you experience such fears, discuss them with your doctor, who should be able to provide medical information that will calm these fears, so tell him or her about your thoughts during your check-ups. Doctors are used to prospective parents being anxious and are usually prepared to answer their questions.

It is also important that you understand the research information available regarding IVF and the incidence of abnormalities. In the general population, around 2 per cent of all babies are born with some type of abnormality. To date, studies of IVF-conceived babies have shown no conclusive evidence that the risk of abnormality is particularly high compared with babies conceived naturally. In a useful fact sheet, 'Risks and complications of assisted conception', the British Fertility Society report that more than one million IVF births worldwide have resulted in an overall abnormality rate that, at 2.6 per cent, is slightly higher than the average.[2] So the risk of abnormality is still very low, will be likely to be less if pre-implantation genetic testing has been carried out and will also be reduced if the mother is younger than thirty-five.

If you are particularly worried, you must discuss your concerns with your doctor, who can advise you on the tests that are available to reassure you. Before taking the tests, discuss with your partner what action you would take if an abnormality were detected. Some couples would not terminate a pregnancy if an abnormality were detected and so feel testing is not necessary. You may worry about the risk of invasive tests such as amniocentesis. However, recent studies show no increased risk of pregnancy loss after the test.[3] If you opt for this test, ensure an experienced specialist carries out the procedure. You can ask for details of the number of these procedures the doctor has undertaken if you are concerned.

Some mothers-to-be are highly anxious about a baby's welfare, even if tests have shown nothing wrong. A woman may be anxious anyway if her own mother had problems during pregnancy, anxiety that can be passed on from mother to daughter. In this case, counselling can help her to enunciate her fears, receive help in challenging these fears and feel supported. She may also feel closer to the baby and more reassured if she finds out its sex, as it is easier to visualise her baby as real and therefore as normal.

What about my age?

It is very common for parents over forty, who discover they are pregnant with their first child, to have an attack of anxiety over their ability to cope with the physical aspects of pregnancy and the emotional considerations of becoming parents. Common fears include 'What if I become ill while my child is still very young?' or 'Am I being selfish wanting a baby when I'm more set in my ways and less flexible?' Older parents also worry that their own parents are elderly, can no longer support the new family as they would wish and are less likely to be a big part of their grandchild's life. If you are concerned about parenting in your forties, tackle these fears before conception rather than leaving them to fester and cause undue anxiety after your child is born.

Arrange for helpers to assist you in caring for elderly and unwell parents so the burden is not on you alone. Pregnancy and parenting are very tough and you will not always have the time or energy to care for both the old and the young. If you do not have other family around, investigate more formal sources of support by contacting your local community services department. Find role models to act as mothering and fathering figures. Elderly parents who are dependent on you are not always able to provide the support new parents need. Identify other couples among your family and friends who can 'mentor' you through early parenting.

Parents often name their own parents as the legal guardians of their children in the event of a tragedy. For older parents, this may not be an option. Instead, siblings or close friends may be suitable. Whoever you choose, talk it over with them before making any legal moves.

Have realistic expectations about yourselves as parents. No matter what your age, at times you are going to be exasperated with the major life changes brought by a baby and you may not have the energy to play rough and tumble ten hours a day. Frustration and exhaustion are normal. Looking after yourselves is even more important if you no longer have the bounce-back ability of a twenty-five-year-old. It is even more important to eat well, exercise and lose unwanted weight. Also take a look at your work values and see where you can achieve a better work/life balance.

There are definitely positives in parenting in your forties. Mature parents generally have a more down-to-earth, realistic outlook on life and greater financial security. Also, at this age many people are much more at ease with themselves, which leads to a more positive self-image for their children. For information about parenting over forty, contact the British organisation Mothers Over Forty (see Useful Contacts, page 201).

Depression in pregnancy

For some mothers-to-be, the anxiety of infertility and IVF gives way to feelings of physical and mental exhaustion, insomnia and the belief that nothing will go right after a positive pregnancy test is announced. It is as if the mind has used up all of its strength to cope with IVF and now there is nothing left. Depression is not uncommon in mothers-to-be — about 10 per cent of all pregnant women experience it — but there is some anecdotal evidence that this is a greater risk for those using IVF.

A diagnosis of depression is made when feelings of sadness, irritability, exhaustion, insomnia, helplessness and loss of pleasure in normal activities have occurred continuously for two weeks. Women who sense they may be experiencing depression need to be evaluated by a professional and treated promptly. If you are experiencing symptoms and believe you are depressed, see your family doctor immediately for a referral to a counselling professional experienced in helping mothers-to-be. You can assess your state of mind and the possibility of depression using questionnaires available on the internet; see Useful Contacts, page 201.

Depression in pregnancy can be fully treated. If help is sought promptly, the condition will not interfere with birth and early parenting. However, leaving the condition untreated will raise the risk of post-natal depression after the birth; finding help quickly is, therefore, important. Also remember that depression is an illness, not a problem to be ashamed of. Having depression in pregnancy does not indicate a mother will not care for her child very well.

Depression in pregnancy should be treated in a holistic way, looking at the mother, her partner, their environment and their histories, both before they met and afterwards. Every woman is different and treatment must be tailored to fit her needs and those of her family.

The most important factor in depression is her history as a child and her own mother's experiences of mothering her. It is amazing how frequently a woman's issues in pregnancy reflect those of her own mother at the same stages in pregnancy. For example, I often find that a woman can recount her mother talking of huge pressures when she was pregnant, such as the father being made redundant or the death of a parent. Jessica's mother, who can remember feeling distraught and exhausted during pregnancy after her father died suddenly, did not realise she needed support, especially as professional help was not readily available at the time. Her anxiety and depression was felt by Jessica when she was in the womb and later newly born. In this instance, Jessica was encouraged to talk to her mother about these experiences, and then to discuss these experiences with me. We talked about how her mother should have been treated and how this would have helped Jessica. With this insight, she could see more clearly why her mother had been in pain, but also how time had helped to ease this pain. Jessica also came to realise how important it was for her unborn baby that she care for herself as much as she could.

Depression in pregnancy can also be traced back to the couples' own parents having poor relationships at the time of pregnancy and birth. Both Craig and Angela, who conceived through IVF, had witnessed their parents separating when they were very small. Angela, particularly, was able to describe feeling alone and unsafe as a very small child when she witnessed her parents yelling at each other and her father walking out on occasions. So both partners came to pregnancy and prospective parenthood feeling unsafe about their own relationship in case they experienced the same problems that had arisen with their own parents.

I often find a mother-to-be who fears relationship problems presents with depression. She feels unable to do anything about her fears when she is pregnant and then comes to feel helpless. Treatment for Angela involved her and Craig learning to talk openly about their childhood experiences and how they felt about them. We then examined their own relationship and explored their satisfactions and issues that arose. Through communicating, they could see they were both projecting their childhood experiences on to their own relationship, making it more likely they would have problems. We worked on improving emotional intimacy by helping each to listen to the other without feeling he or she had to 'fix' anything. The couple also discovered the value of times of quiet when they could be together.

Another cause of depression in pregnancy, particularly for a mother who has had to cope with infertility and IVF, is the absence of her own mother. Today families often live far from each other. For the most part, it has little effect. A woman may miss her parents but cope well. During pregnancy, however, this ability to cope often disintegrates.

Karen had moved cities after marriage, far from her parents. Although she made frequent trips to see them, she enjoyed her working and social life in her new location. Her mother came to visit during IVF treatment to give her support. But after Karen discovered her pregnancy, her mother became ill. Not only was her mother prevented from coming to help out, but Karen lost her main confidant because her mother struggled to hold a conversation at times. Karen failed to realise how much she missed her mother and felt guilty for wanting to talk about herself. She slipped into depression, feeling tearful and distressed even at work.

Through counselling, Karen came to understand that her need to be with her mother was normal and not something to feel guilty about. She learned a way to talk to her husband and to garner further support from him while her mother was less available. Karen had regular sessions with me so that she could let out her feelings, thereby releasing tension and helping her feel less depressed. We also focused her attention on an older friend who lived only twenty minutes away, had children and was a good support for her. By the time her mother had recovered, Karen was much happier and carried on using her new supports even after the mother-daughter conversations resumed.

For more serious cases of depression, medication may sometimes be recommended, particularly if the mother-to-be has experienced a previous episode of depression requiring medication. Modern anti-depressants have far fewer side effects than the older style drugs, and there are medications that research has indicated are safe in pregnancy. Although it is recommended that pregnant women avoid medication, in each case it is necessary to weigh up the pros and cons of such treatment. A seriously depressed mother fares much better taking medication that keeps her safe rather than feeling she cannot survive.

It is also important to note that prospective fathers can suffer depression too. The signs are seeming especially irritable, exhausted, having problems sleeping and finding pleasure hard to find. Seeking a referral to a male counsellor or psychologist can help the man find support and strategies to cope with this stressful time of life.

As pregnancy progresses

As IVF parents move into the second and third trimesters, issues they face change. Most describe passing the three-month period with great relief because the risk of miscarriage has significantly decreased. However, the anxiety rarely goes completely, and they appear to have lost much of the 'innocence' that first-time parents-to-be often show, that wide-eyed wonder and excitement.

The second trimester is the time to focus on good self-care, to strengthen the relationship and to balance life as much as possible. Time taken to relax, organise and relate well will reap huge rewards in the months to come. This is the time when the woman is likely to feel less tired and nauseous and will be able to resume a more normal life. The man, who often feels fairly helpless if his partner is exhausted and nauseous all the time, will enjoy being able to engage in a more normal relationship.

One of the common issues in IVF pregnancies is the concern over the mother 'doing the right thing' by her baby. All pregnant women worry to a degree about what they eat, drink, how much sleep they have, how stressed they get and how much or how little exercise they take. With the longing for a pregnancy that has been a feature of life for some time, IVF couples tend to worry that much more. At times the mother-to-be may feel she is not the perfect woman she feels she should be after being given the wonderful gift of pregnancy. The prospective father may be over-cautious with his partner. Sensible advice for both includes knowing the risks in pregnancy, taking precautions to avoid risks and learning to better manage recurring worries.

Medical check-ups are vital for all pregnant women. You will suffer less anxiety if you ensure you attend all your regular checks and have regular blood and urine tests. Generally, IVF pregnancy risks are the same as those for any pregnancy, although there are two issues that are very slightly more prevalent after IVF conception.

Pre-eclampsia, which affects 2 to 10 per cent of all pregnancies, is a serious condition. Research shows a greater risk of pre-eclampsia when parents are older or have experienced infertility.[4] Pre-eclampsia can be detected promptly with urine tests and blood pressure readings.

Researchers in Sweden have also found a slightly elevated risk of a condition termed placenta praevia for IVF pregnancies.[5] This condition occurs where the placenta covers part of the cervix, blocking the baby's progress through the birth canal. Some believe that the introduction of embryos into the womb after test-tube fertilisation may increase the likelihood of implantation lower down in the womb, which causes placenta praevia. This problem often results in bleeding during pregnancy, as well as increasing the risk of a premature birth. Any bleeding should be investigated promptly, although it is not uncommon in assisted pregnancies and may not be serious. Blood tests and ultrasound examinations can assess where the placenta is lying. The condition, if it appears, will be monitored closely and a caesarean section is usually performed.

Implantation of more than one embryo increases the risk of multiple pregnancies, and as many as 23 per cent of couples conceiving through IVF carry more than one baby. It has long been known that multiple pregnancies pose greater risks for the mother and babies than a single pregnancy. A multiple pregnancy does not have to mean the woman has to lie down for nine months, but doctors generally warn against strenuous exercise. Mothers-to-be often feel extremely fatigued in the second and third trimesters and will need plenty of rest. Those carrying multiples will also need to avoid unnecessary strain, intense fatigue and possible early deliveries. Both partners should talk over these issues with their doctor and with the woman's employer if appropriate. For more information on multiple pregnancy, consult Rachel Franklin's book *Expecting Twins, Triplets and More: A Doctor's Guide to a Happy and Healthy Multiple Pregnancy.*

Every pregnant woman needs to be aware of the risk of contracting toxoplasmosis, and should take care to avoid contamination, particularly if she has pets. Precautions include: cooking meat until it is no longer pink; avoiding unpasturised milk, milk products and uncooked cured meats; washing fruit and vegetables thoroughly; washing hands before meals; avoiding cleaning litter trays, which should be cleaned daily with disinfectant and boiling water.

Both partners need to understand the risks inherent in the pregnancy, agree on precautions to take and then be mindful that over-worry can become a habit. Avoid getting angry with a partner who worries too much; instead, stay calm and provide reassurance.

For parents who are particularly anxious about their unborn baby and who only feel reassured by medical check-ups, seeing an ultrasound picture or hearing a heartbeat and having a foetal doppler at home to record the baby's heart beat would be wise. These machines can be bought or rented from a number of specialist medical companies. Get advice about using these machines from your medical practitioner.

Other concerns that IVF couples have raised are about travelling abroad and flying. Having holidays before the baby is born is a good idea and there is no evidence to show flying and high altitude have any effects on pregnancy until the very late stages of the third trimester. The main concern is to avoid countries where there is a threat of disease: check with your doctor and the government's foreign affairs department website. In addition, pregnant women need to listen to their own feelings and only travel where and when they feel comfortable. I have talked to mothers who have taken trips they were not confident about during pregnancy, only to spend the next few months in a state of high anxiety, worrying they may have inadvertently hurt their baby. Finally, pregnant women should avoid sunbathing or hot spas: both can lead to over-heating, which is not advisable in pregnancy.

Complementary therapies in later pregnancy

Great care must be taken by pregnant women seeking to use complementary therapies. But there are well-researched benefits from certain techniques. Consult your obstetrician about the suitability of the therapy for your specific needs before going ahead. It is essential to find a practitioner who holds suitable qualifications in the speciality; always ask to see professional credentials before beginning the first therapy session.

Most researched is pregnancy massage. A group of medical and psychological experts at the University of Miami's Touch Research Institute have conducted studies on the benefits of massage, for both mother and baby and have shown that pregnancy massage decreases anxiety levels and stress hormone concentrations in mothers, in addition to lowering the rates of premature birth.[6, 7] These benefits are well worth bearing in mind because prematurity is more common in IVF pregnancies. Opting for a regular program of massage throughout the pregnancy can provide significant benefits to an IVF mother and baby. There is nothing to stop the prospective father enjoying the benefits of massage therapy himself in order to remain calm.

Another gentle healing technique available to IVF parents is reiki. This non-invasive Japanese technique is in the early stages of use in medical research; however, preliminary studies show that the therapy significantly decreases depression and anxiety and relieves pain, which can make it suitable to use when giving birth. It involves a reiki master using simple hands-on, gentle-touch and visualisation techniques, with the goal of improving the flow of life energy in a person. Once attuned, you can use your hands to give reiki to yourself or to others. Anecdotal evidence suggests that men using reiki on their partners can increase the bond between him and the unborn child. It may also relieve his sense of helplessness. Addresses of reiki centres can be found on the internet.

Relating as a couple

The second trimester and the early stage of the third is a great time for IVF couples to regain the emotional intimacy of the days before fertility issues overwhelmed their lives: joy in being together, sharing of common interests and having fun together. I have found most couples moving through IVF have lost this intimacy. Regaining it requires some extra effort, but the benefits to both partners and to their unborn child are enormous.

At this stage of the pregnancy, I ask couples to reflect on their first years as a couple and remember the times that were the most enjoyable. They may remember visiting museums and antique shops, going for walks, frequenting bookstores and watching movies. I suggest they try to fit one of these activities into each week, taking turns to organise the event. This time together works wonders in bringing couples emotionally closer together. The activities also prompt memories of earlier, less stressful times and a shifting of focus from the IVF procedures. The couple also regain a sense that life can be ordinary and fun.

If mid-pregnancy brings an emotional distance between you both, there are a few alternative ideas to try. You may benefit from relationship counselling. A therapist can help you explore your feelings towards each other and the reasons for the emotional distance in a safe environment, as well as providing you with techniques to try to increase the positive side of your relationship.

Another simple but powerful technique is to change the attention given to your partner. In times of stress, we often feel sensitive and react poorly to a comment our partner makes that inadvertently hurts us. When this happens repeatedly, it is easy to focus on the bad aspects of our partner and this only leads to emotional distance. If you find yourselves focusing only on the tensions between you, you can change your thinking by re-focusing your attention on the things your partner does to make you feel good. Ensure you compliment your partner when he or she is loving, helpful or thoughtful and ignore anything that hurts you. This technique requires patience and practise but will lead to more positive interactions between you and consequently a more intimate relationship.

Reviewing finances

One thing that can weigh heavily on the mind in pregnancy, yet is rarely discussed, is money.

If a couple have reviewed their finances before beginning IVF treatment and have made plans to cope with the additional costs, they will be in a much better position during pregnancy. Couples who have not done their financial homework, however, often begin to panic at this point, realising they have little room to manoeuvre.

Ideally, having a little spare money and low debt levels is a great position to be in. Some mothers-to-be find the stress of IVF and pregnancy leave them needing to cut down their working hours and/or finish work earlier than they had intended. A little financial freedom gives a couple this option. This is particularly true for women who experience bleeding, those who suffer great anxiety and those with multiple pregnancies.

Couples who have not been able to organise their finances before pregnancy will find that mid-pregnancy provides another opportunity to visit this very necessary task. Find a reputable financial planner through a professional body or visit some of the useful financial planning websites: they often include guides to budgeting and dealing with unexpected events, information about how to manage the loans taken out for treatment together with mortgages and normal household payments.

Shopping for the baby

Many couples begin buying items for their baby towards the end of the second trimester, but if the baby was conceived through IVF, they may be far more cautious, frightened to buy anything for their unborn baby for fear of somehow jinxing the pregnancy. In this instance, go with these feelings until you reach twenty-eight to thirty weeks of pregnancy.

Although babies conceived through IVF are more likely to be born a little early, buying just the essential items at this time should work well. A bassinet, pram, car capsule, baby carrier (sling), bottles and steriliser, bedding, baby suits and vests, baby monitor, nappies and muslins are the only items parents will need immediately.

If you are pregnant with twins or triplets, you may well go into labour early but would not need equipment at home immediately: most multiple babies spend at least a week in hospital. Your need for equipment will be greater, of course, and therefore your costs higher if you are expecting multiples, so investigate borrowing some equipment from friends or acquiring things second-hand. And ask the advice of other parents of multiples to ensure that you do not spend money on non-essential items; if you do not know any, join a multiple birth association and register to join its online forum where you can question other parents (see Useful Contacts, page 201).

The baby shower

Baby showers evoke mixed responses from all pregnant mothers. There are those who really enjoy the celebration and who may mark the end of work before going on maternity leave with a baby shower. Other women do not want too much fuss and are happy just for very close friends and relatives to offer emotional support and perhaps small gifts.

Women carrying babies conceived through IVF also have varying feelings. For those still fearing something going wrong, it is advisable to tell close friends and family that you would like to have a baby shower just after the baby is born. You may also like to let people know you would much rather they keep gifts to give to you until after the birth. If you fear offending anyone, let a relative or close friend tell those around you that you have fears that would be exacerbated by gift-giving and, instead, you would much prefer this way of celebrating.

Parents of multiples may also opt for a shower well after birth. Couples know they are much more likely to give birth prematurely if they are expecting more than one baby and the stress of a party may be too much to cope with.

5

The Birth

From the moment we saw our babies, we fell in love with them.

'It was all very surreal until I had that date booked, then reality hit home,' reports a woman who gave birth to her IVF baby by caesarean section after doctors discovered a low-lying placenta. 'I thought, in five weeks I'm going to be a mum. That's when the whole huge process, the waiting, the nerves, everything, became secondary to the fact I was having a real live baby. Was I scared? I certainly was!' The last part of the pregnancy, from week thirty to the birth, marks an important time for parents to prepare physically and emotionally, for both the process of birth and for the early days of parenting.

About the baby

All parents need to know what their baby is capable of before she arrives in the world. This helps them prepare to begin caring for her. Having conceived by IVF, your need for information is even greater, as this will help you come to the birth feeling able to parent in a relaxed manner.

From the twenty-eighth week, most couples begin to focus more on their baby and her characteristics. Babies born beyond this time generally do well and so couples feel some sense of reassurance in reaching this milestone. This time is a good stage to begin to focus on the amazing skills your unborn baby possesses.

By twenty-eight weeks' gestation, your baby's eyes can open and she can see shades of light and dark. She can hear your heartbeat, other body sounds and muffled voices around her. She can distinguish mum's voice from others and will often quieten in response to mum talking. She begins to lose the fine hair that has covered her body, she is able to feel pain and her lungs are becoming ready to take over the job of providing oxygen.

Babies at this stage are very responsive to stress as mum's stress hormones released into the body travel across the placenta. Many mums report an unborn baby doing somersaults in response to a big fright. For this reason, the last weeks of pregnancy are a good time for both prospective parents to have a quiet relaxing time together. Playing relaxation or classical music in the evening or giving mum a foot massage are great ways to help baby feel relaxed and safe too! Since a baby at this stage can recognise familiar sounds, using the same pieces of music played again can help increase the relaxation as the familiarity provides a cue for the brain to de-stress. You can use just the same pieces of music to play once baby is born if she has an unsettled, fretful period as all babies inevitably do.

About the prospective parents

Anxieties parents may have had on and off throughout the pregnancy rarely go away at this point, just before birth. Many women report feeling anxious about their unborn babies, fearing they are moving less than they should. A first-time mother is particularly anxious, as she has no reference point to tell her what is normal for a healthy unborn baby.

If you are first-time parents, you may be given kick charts to complete each day as part of your antenatal care. Generally, you tick off your baby's first ten kicks and note when they have been felt. You may have ten by early morning or by the end of the day: movements vary day to day and from one baby to the next. As yet, there is no conclusive evidence to suggest kick charts work to protect the baby — and no evidence to show that they do not help. If you are asked to complete them, it is usually helpful to do so.

You can also reassure yourself of your baby's well-being by noting down his typical movement patterns in a day. Perhaps he is always busy when you go to bed at night, or when you sit down for a tea break mid-morning. Exercise may make him sleepy and quiet and he may have a busier period when you wake in the morning. Knowing his typical patterns can alert you to any changes in his routine. Your intuition is a very valuable diagnostic tool: if you feel he has changed his behaviour, contact your doctor for advice. The father's role here is to support his partner by listening to her concerns and acting upon them. It rarely helps to tell a mother-to-be, 'There's nothing wrong.' Without evidence, this comment often makes her even more anxious as she is not being taken seriously. Instead, if you have an anxious partner reporting movement changes, focus her attention on the kick patterns, the heartbeat if you have a doppler (see page 73), and on getting to see the doctor if there are concerns over either of these two measures of the baby's well-being. The more you listen and act on your partner's feelings, the safer she will feel.

Another aspect of the last weeks of pregnancy where a man can play an important role is in helping his partner care for herself. During the last ten weeks, the baby is growing in length and putting on weight at a rapid rate; consequently, the mother can feel very tired. This is when it is easy to pile on unwanted weight by craving sweet foods. Anxiety about the birth and early parenting can also lead to comfort eating which can have an adverse effect on weight and mum's self-esteem after the birth. So it is important at times of craving to turn to foods that supply good nutrients without a lot of calories. There are also foods that contain naturally occurring mood stabilising chemicals which can help aid anxiety. These foods include oats, white meat and dairy products and a partner can be of help by suggesting just such a healthy alternative to sweet foods.

A pregnant mother needs plenty of rest in the last ten weeks but also some light exercise such as a short walk, unless her doctor advises against it. Talk to your medical practitioner about how much exercise is sensible and use this as a basis for a daily plan leading up to the birth.

Both partners need to be involved in ensuring their workload is not too great — and in the decision about when the woman will stop work. The timing can be earlier than the original date set if she is struggling to cope or there are medical reasons.

A few expectant mothers try to keep working as close to their due date as possible. They may come to birth and early parenting somewhat ill prepared if they have not had the time to reflect on what has happened through conception and pregnancy and what will come after the birth. If you are a mother-to-be needing to work close to your due date, even with reduced hours, make sure you take the time out to relax and to plan the resources to help you cope with early parenting.

Occasionally, a woman will keep working to avoid her fears of the birth and the early weeks of being a mother. Occasionally, it may be the father who does the long hours, taking on more work to avoid having the time to think about becoming a father. This tactic does not decrease anxiety in the long-term and can result in sizeable panic when labour begins. If you or your partner shows signs of being unable to confront the birth and its aftermath, arrange to see a counsellor through your doctor, hospital or birthing centre.

Ready to parent?

First-time parents will be invited to attend antenatal classes at their chosen hospital or birthing centre, to help them prepare for the birth. Classes generally cover the stages of labour, pain relief, breathing and muscle control and sometimes basic newborn care. Second-time parents, who have had a sizeable gap in between babies, may feel reassured by attending classes again; alternatively, there is an online refresher course (see Useful Contacts, page 201).

Antenatal classes are valuable to help parents prepare physically and mentally for birth. However, they tend to focus all of the attention on the birthing process. Many new parents say they were so focused on that one day they had no idea what to do next. This is where psychological preparation for early parenting can be of immense help. I run a session for parents-to-be about six to eight weeks before the baby's due date, or a few weeks earlier for multiple babies. This is to encourage the couple to focus on the changes they are about to make, moving from independent people to new parenthood.

The session generally follows a pattern, one that parents can adopt at home. We start by each partner describing their happiest memory of their childhood; this helps each get in touch with him or herself as a child, an important part of becoming a healthy, happy parent. I then ask each partner to describe two aspects of their own parents' parenting that they would want to pass on to their child. Answers may include feeling respected by their parents, loving their problem-solving skills, feeling the hours a parent spent helping them master school was important or valuing the routines of life parents put in place to help them feel safe. Often, these memories have not been shared between the partners before and it is a moving and powerful time. The next focus is on the difficulties each partner had with aspects of their parents' actions. This is not meant to be 'parent-bashing'; instead, it is simply a reflection on the hurts of childhood and how we may parent differently to minimise our children's hurts. The aim is to create a new generation of parents more sensitive to their children's needs than the last. Many report difficulties with criticism, parents who were too busy keeping the family financially afloat to be emotionally available, and those who put enormous pressure on their children to perform academically or in some other way. This exercise helps parents-to-be focus on how they would like to change old ideas for more empathic parenting. It also helps couples to understand their partner's need to perhaps avoid criticism or provide a more rounded education.

For parents who have already had a child, I hold a session focusing on their experiences during the birth and the first six weeks of being parents. Many parents remember the first six weeks of parenting as being chaotic, extremely stressful and a time they do not wish to repeat. To create a better experience the second time around, we look at each partner's concerns: perhaps feeding took a long time to establish, the baby may have been hard to settle, or perhaps there was resentment that the father could not take more time off work. I then help the couple focus on strategies to meet these problems if they happen again, assisting partners to identify supports they can use outside of the relationship, including parents, siblings, other relatives and friends. I teach basic sleep and settling techniques (see pages 104–05), reassuring both partners that there are gentle ways to help a newborn settle more easily. We look at schedules so partners can share the care in more appropriate ways and are able to talk to each other without blaming the other if they are struggling. Once this session is complete, parents generally feel much better prepared to meet their new baby.

Developing a birth plan

A birth plan is a document, drawn up by prospective parents, which seeks to address some of the choices they may be asked to make during the birth.

It helps to alert health professionals to the specific needs of the family at a time when the partners may be ill-equipped to explain their needs aloud.

Asking mothers about their ideas regarding a birth plan will provide enough answers to fill a book. Fathers often look confused at the mention of a birth plan. Some new mothers and fathers swear their birth plan kept them going and made them realise they could give birth naturally. There are also new parents who are shocked by the birth and feel the planning process was a waste of time because they felt so out of control. Still others say that considering the options helped, but nothing went exactly as planned. My own view is that it is essential to be realistic about the fact you do not know what to expect; nevertheless, the planning process certainly has its place in helping a couple prepare physically and emotionally for the birth of their IVF-conceived baby.

A good birth plan is all about options: what is possible, what is desired and what may happen. For first-time parents, prior planning introduces some of the choices they may have to make and helps them consider the strong feelings they may have about aspects of giving birth. If this is a second or third baby, parents can build their plan on what happened last time.

Many couples want to establish some control over a process that seems alien and even frightening. This is particularly so for couples who have felt out of control through a diagnosis of infertility and who have undergone IVF treatment. If you require control, planning can help you become informed but it cannot control a process that is different for every family. However, planning can make you feel you have choices — and this can help you no matter what the birth process brings.

The first piece of information you need for your birth plan is to explain how your baby was conceived. This will help the professionals who care for you to understand your feelings and your need for good information. Obstetricians, midwives and paediatricians are becoming more knowledgeable about the particular needs of families created through IVF and will react better to your questions and requests if they are briefed about your treatment.

The first decision that is made and noted on the birth plan is the desired method of giving birth. A number of studies highlighted in *Progress in Reproductive Medicine* recently demonstrated that the method of delivery is often different for IVF and non-IVF mums. The normal caesarean rate for non-IVF pregnancies worldwide is about 20 per cent of all deliveries. The authors Asch and Studd report a worldwide caesarean rate for IVF pregnancies of 35–58 per cent. As yet, there are no definite reasons for the discrepancy, however anxiety on the part of the parents may often be a factor in addition to medical practitioners deciding to use caution with an IVF pregnancy. It is also true that older mothers are more likely to have a caesarean for both IVF and non-IVF conceived babies.

Your doctor may advise you a caesarean section is preferable or even essential due to placenta praevia, a multiple pregnancy, a breech pregnancy, concerns about the baby, or if you go into premature labour. Most parents are happy to consider this option if medical wisdom suggests it is the safest method.

A number of mothers, particularly those in their late thirties and forties, feel that a caesarean would be 'easier'. In some circumstances, this is a reaction to the anxiety they have over their unborn baby and the feeling that birth would be safer if controlled by a doctor. In reality, evidence suggests that a normal delivery is safer for the baby if there are no medical complications: it may be safer because a vaginal birth naturally triggers instinctive breathing in a newborn.

If you are concerned about the lack of control apparent in a normal delivery, it is important to discuss your concerns with your doctor or midwife. The professionals who guide you through birth can make additional arrangements to help you cope with anxiety, perhaps by requesting foetal monitoring at regular intervals or even continuously during labour.

A visit to the hospital or birthing centre is a good way to allay some of the fears about the birth. It is a good idea to familiarise yourselves with the layout of the unit, the location of the car park, the visitors' waiting areas and the labour ward or theatres. Meeting one or two staff members as you visit is also reassuring.

For mothers with single pregnancies, packing a hospital bag around thirty-four weeks is a good idea even if the bag 'hangs around' for a while. You have a one in ten chance of going into labour prematurely, so good preparation will help reduce your fears of not being ready. For multiple pregnancies, have a bag packed from thirty weeks just in case because there is a very significant risk of early delivery. Also note that having a baby a little prematurely does not automatically mean disaster: plenty of babies are born at thirty-five or thirty-six weeks with no major problems.

The packing of a bag is, in itself, a form of psychological preparation. Take time to plan what to take and pack the essentials such as nightclothes, dressing gown, slippers, toiletries, nipple cream, maternity pads and possibly disposable briefs, nappies, nappy change cream and baby clothes. It is a good idea to remember a change of clothes for going home from hospital (men rarely find the right items to bring in, being so stressed about bringing the new family home). Also think of a few treats, such as facial wipes and a soothing facial moisturiser, a good hand cream and shampoo. If you are planning a normal delivery, include any items you wish to use while you are in labour, such as a sponge to cool you, aromatherapy oils, your birth plan of course and perhaps a relaxation tape or two. Also keep telephone numbers of friends, family, neighbours and other helpers handy.

Once the hospital bag is planned, both parents need to turn their thoughts to the types of pain relief they may wish to use, as well as any options they feel strongly about not having. If you are planning for a caesarean delivery, note that most are performed under spinal or epidural anaesthesia, but a general anaesthetic is also an option if you are very frightened or have reacted poorly to an epidural or spinal previously. The disadvantage of a general anaesthetic is that you will not be able to meet your baby immediately, and some mothers feel the bonding takes longer to establish if there has been separation. One IVF mother experienced this disappointment: 'I wanted a natural birth in the birth centre. I ended up with a c-section under a general and didn't see my babies for three hours after they were born.'

For a planned vaginal delivery, there are a number of pain relief options. You may opt for a full epidural, particularly if you are in labour for a long time, or a low-dose epidural that allows you the possibility of moving around. You can elect to have an injection of a painkiller such as pethidine or you can breathe nitrous oxide.

You may also opt to use natural pain relief techniques to supplement other methods. Hypnotherapy is particularly effective in reducing the pain reported by labouring mothers and the need for stronger pain relief.[1] Hypnotherapy needs to be learned for a period before you can use it during childbirth. The process allows you to alter your state of consciousness to experience a 'daydreaming' sensation that brings feelings of safety and relaxation, both of which are very valuable to those who have been through IVF procedures. Hypnotherapy is best taught by a suitably quali-fied medical practitioner or psychologist. Ensure you consult a practitioner experienced in helping parents-to-be and encourage the father to learn the technique for moments during the birth when he too feels very stressed.

Another pain relief technique is the use of music. The anaesthesiologist Fred Schwarz practises music medicine, the use of familiar tunes to reduce the need for chemical pain relief.[2] Dr Schwarz suggests several significant benefits of music for couples going through both vaginal and caesarean deliveries: firstly, music decreases the anxiety caused by the unfamiliar surroundings; secondly, a choice of music gives the couple a chance to exert control over aspects of the birth, and, finally, music can speed up labour and decrease pain for both types of deliveries by slowing the breathing rate. Music that has been played during pregnancy can also soothe a newborn, who will recognise sounds heard in the womb. Soothing meditation music or classical pieces are particularly good for childbirth.

Support people to assist during labour and birth are also important considerations when you develop your birth plan. Some people are particularly good in stressful situations: they are able to stay calm and focused and keep their own emotions at bay. Others are temperamentally more affected by stress and less able to keep emotions in check. Talk to each other about how you each deal with stress and ensure you avoid blaming or 'pointing the finger' at your partner for not coping in a way you would like. Talk about how you have helped each other in stressful situations previously and what events have not been easy to cope with. Consider whether you are able to give each other the support needed or whether it would be useful to have other support people: mothers, siblings or friends.

If there are no suitable family members or close friends to act as couple supports during delivery, some couples consider using a doula. A doula is a specially trained and professional birth assistant who establishes a relationship with the couple before birth and later attends the birth to assist mum and dad in coping. For parents coping with the anxieties of IVF, pregnancy and birth, having a doula assist during childbirth can be a wonderful (and not necessarily expensive) option to calm fears and provide a more positive birth experience.

A doula can be present whatever delivery method you opt for. She is trained in childbirth education and may have additional qualifications in breastfeeding support and massage. Some doulas can also be available for a few weeks after birth to help establish breastfeeding and a good bond between mum, dad and baby. Further information about doulas is available on the internet and the addresses are given in the 'Useful Contacts' section of the book.

The next step in the planning process is to consider any options you are adamant you do not want to use. You must make these clear. Examples include drugs you do not want, continuous foetal monitoring if you wish to move about during labour, or trainee health-care professionals assisting. You may wish to highlight your desire to avoid a caesarean if possible and your wish to try for a natural delivery.

The birth plan should also include decisions you want to make in advance of the birth itself. You may wish to have a vaginally delivered baby put straight on to your belly, you may wish for a caesarean baby to remain with the father at all times, you may want the father to cut the cord. If you wish to circumcise a boy also note this on your plan.

An example birth plan is shown below:

Birth plan for Barbara Dickson

Hospital/centre: North Shore Hospital

Planned delivery method: Normal/caesarean section

Date (if planned): N/a

Conception: Our baby was conceived using IVF. We are naturally anxious after all we have been through.

Pain management: We prefer to try for a water birth.

Options we may consider: Nitrous oxide, epidural if necessary.

Alternative pain relief methods: Hypnotherapy, music therapy.

Support people:

For delivery: My partner, mother and doula.

At the hospital/centre: Siblings, parents.

Baby monitoring: Continuous, or intermittent if we are anxious.

Special requests during birth: A quiet room, no observers, CD player with our choice of music.

Special requests immediately after birth: Father to cut the cord, delivery on to mother's stomach, father to accompany our baby at all times.

Home births

The safety of home births compared with hospital births remains a highly contentious issue. Major considerations for a decision about where to give birth focus on the progress of the pregnancy to date and whether there have been complications. Professionals may also look at previous births the mother has been through to calculate the possibility of unforseen difficulties.

If after IVF treatment you are pregnant with multiples or have had any complications in pregnancy, you will be advised to give birth in hospital. If pregnancy has been uneventful, a birthing centre may be an option if your doctor or midwife supports this.

There are no data as yet for home births for IVF-conceived babies. My own opinion is that the probably small but not-yet quantifiable elevation in birth abnormalities for assisted pregnancies, combined with the additional anxiety most parents naturally experience, makes hospital a better option. However, you can have choices even if a hospital birth is deemed necessary: you are free to visit several hospitals so you can talk to staff and see their facilities.

A new parents' survival guide

Before the birth, couples are better prepared for the transition to parenthood if they can make tentative plans for the six weeks after the baby arrives. If no thought has been given to this time, the anxiety IVF brings, mixed with the sleep deprivation that comes with most newborns, can create a traumatic time for all concerned.

I recommend IVF parents make a survival plan for the first six weeks of parenting, just as they prepared a birth plan. A very useful part of a survival plan is the availability of a computer, which offers many stress-reducing techniques, including grocery shopping from home, communicating with friends when the telephone is impossible and requesting help from breastfeeding organisations and others you may need to contact for help. (If parents are not computer-literate, a friend may teach them the basics or they can take a quick course; second-hand computers can be picked up very cheaply, and the internet is widely available.)

Another essential part of any six-week survival plan is a good family doctor on hand. As you have been through IVF treatment, you probably already have a sympatheic family doctor, but check whether she or he wishes to provide baby care or can recommend a colleague with more experience in this field. You need an empathic and reassuring family doctor, who you can see quickly and will take your concerns about your baby seriously. Talk to any local mothers you know: most will have strong views on who would be a good family doctor for you.

Also investigate the nearest children's hospital and check if they have a hotline for parents. Many do, providing wonderful reassurance for anxious new parents.

Attach your survival guide to the fridge well before your due date so that you know where to go to get help at times when you are too stressed or too tired to think properly. Creating the guide is also a great way to reduce anxiety. This task will stop you having to rehearse over and over again information you need to remember after the birth.

Here is what a six-week survival guide should include:

Our six-week survival guide

Coming home from hospital: *Who will collect you and help you settle in.*

Assistance with breastfeeding: *[The local breastfeeding asssociation will have a telephone and email service to help you with breastfeeding problems.] Address, telephone number and website.*

Our local child and family health centre: *Name, address and telephone number.*

Family doctor: *Name, address and telephone number.*

Local children's hospital hotline: *Telephone number.*

Nearest children's hospital: *Name, address and telephone number.*

Counselling professional, private midwife, doula: *Names and contact numbers, including emergency contacts.*

Getting food and provisions: *Detail arrangements for a friend to shop for you, or set up an online account at a local supermarket if such a service is available.*

Online baby items: *For items you don't need to leave the house to buy, go to online stores or consider buying second hand online.*

Help in the home: *Consider a fortnightly or weekly cleaner for the early days.*

Premature labour

Prematurity is *not* a factor in all IVF pregnancies; indeed, for single embryo transfers, it appears to be uncommon. For multiple embryo transfers and/ or multiple pregnancies, however, prematurity may be a concern.

Experts believe that the foetus initiates labour and yet we know little about why labour happens prematurely in many cases. Stress may play a role, as well as cervical problems, infections or the presence of more than one foetus. Any sign of labour beginning before thirty-seven weeks requires immediate medical attention and efforts to help the parents cope emotionally.

Some parents know in advance their baby or babies may be born early. If this is the case, there is a great deal that can be done to improve the outcome for all of you. Information is the first priority: ensure you know what is happening with your body and with the foetus. Find out whether rest will help. You may be given steroid injections that can help your baby or babies with their breathing. You can also find information and emotional support from an organisation run by parents of premature babies to help those facing a premature delivery or who have already delivered prematurely (see Useful Contacts, page 201).

As with all births, try to avoid engaging in spiralling negative thoughts. Encourage yourselves not to leap to disastrous conclusions if contractions begin early. Conserve energy by deep breathing and remember the importance of staying calm. Ensure you get to hospital quickly and with someone supporting you. Listen carefully as health-care professionals explain what is happening and what you can do to help yourself and the baby. Unless arrangements have to be made for a speedy delivery, you can talk over your options with staff before making decisions.

Depending on how far advanced it is, you may receive drugs that can put off labour. Bed rest and deep breathing may reduce stress, which in turn can stop or slow down contractions. You may need to remain in hospital for as long as the labour can be held off. This can be a frustrating and very worrying time, a time when keeping a diary each day has proved to be a very positive way of coping for both parents. Accept offers of support at this time, as helping hands offer an emotional boost for both of you. A mother to boy/girl twins born at twenty-five weeks after four weeks of threatened labour reported that she wished she had been able to organise more support for herself and her partner for after the babies were born, when they were visiting the twins every day. 'No one was looking after us,' she explained. 'And there was no one to organise food for us when we got home from the hospital.'

The medical staff will be highly focused during the delivery of a premature baby; parents often feel most alone. Do not be frightened to ask questions, however — your input is very much needed and expressing your feelings helps both of you cope more effectively. You may be asked to avoid certain birth options, such as a vaginal delivery or the injection of painkilling drugs. Always ask for more information if you feel unsure about a particular choice you are asked to make. Review the techniques described earlier to achieve a positive birth, as these can be valuable during a pre-term delivery.

Premature births almost always result in a loss of control for parents, who may feel cheated by the medical intervention required to ensure their baby or babies survive. 'There is less of a feeling that I had done it "naturally",' explained one mother of two sets of twins. In the circumstances, these feelings are very normal and can be relieved by talking them through with a counsellor, as well as by evaluating the options you would have chosen if events had turned out differently. This is part of the 'acceptance process'.

Parents who have been through a pre-term birth need 'special care' too (see pages 106–11). Many parents have said that small events may trigger intense emotional reactions, feelings they had during the day of premature birth and during the weeks of having babies in the neonatal intensive care unit. 'In hospital, just hearing a drip is enough to set me off,' reports one mother who cared for her twins in the NICU for seventeen weeks. These parents can be helped significantly by being allowed to review the birth process with a counsellor, social worker or psychologist.

The birth day

This is a time to focus on the anxiety-reduction strategies and methods of staying calm described earlier. Parents may like to read over this chapter several times in the weeks leading up to the birth so that strategies remain fresh in the mind.

Keeping anxiety at bay will be tough, but it is very much worthwhile because your attitude of mind will have an enormous bearing on how you negotiate the birth of your baby. There are three very powerful anxiety management techniques for achieving a happy birth.

Technique one: deep breathing

In the days leading up to birth and during the process itself, focus on the deep breathing technique that is such a vital part of managing anxiety during birth. This technique involves breathing with your abdomen and chest (see pages 41–42). Remind each other to go back to this form of breathing during stressful parts of the birth process. Deep breathing or 'belly breathing' not only helps the natural process, it will avoid you feeling traumatised, and allows you to think rationally and to digest important information you are given by hospital staff. Deep breathing helps you to conserve energy for the time ahead.

Technique two: talk, don't shut down

A very important part of giving birth in a calm and positive way is that both partners must reveal their feelings to each other and to the staff before they feel overwhelmed. Many parents sense that something is going wrong during the birth process but are too afraid to ask. The feelings of panic and loss of control grow, no one around the couple realises what is happening, and forever after the birth will be remembered as a traumatic and disturbing event, even though nothing difficult may have actually happened.

You will benefit from talking to each other before the birth about how you can signal you need help. The female partner, particularly, will need to be able to indicate to her partner that help is needed quickly, perhaps with a hand signal to avoid the need to talk. Your body may be telling you something feels very wrong, yet a quick reassurance from staff can assure you all is completely normal. If you have not been through the birth process before, you will experience many different feelings that may cause you alarm. The man can use similar strategies to ensure he can attract the attention of a staff member if anxiety is increasing.

Technique three: avoid catastrophising

It seems to be a very human condition to feel something is wrong, then to launch immediately into believing the worst. Some people are prone to thinking situations are far worse than they actually are — something counselling professionals call 'catastrophising'. There are two main problems with this habit: firstly, when parents are already stressed after fertility treatment and pregnancy, the birth process can be extremely frightening if every sensation is interpreted as the worst possible scenario; secondly, constant fear uses up precious energy that parents need to help them move through the birth process.

If you are aware you tend to adopt a negative approach to problems, or if this is the thinking style of your partner, you can gently remind each other that one problem is not the end of the world. Perhaps you need to rely on a forceps-assisted delivery or, after several hours of labour, you feel you need pain relief even though you wished not to use this; be clear that a change in plan is only that. Focus on the aspects of the birth that are going according to plan and try to believe a change in the plan does not mean a loss of control or the end of a happy birth. There are many other factors that can make sure your baby arrives safely and joyfully.

Now we are a family

The baby has arrived. The initial flurry of shock and excitement has passed. Family and friends have been to visit the new arrival. Now parents find themselves left literally 'holding the baby'. This is the time when the enormity of the changes in their lives often hits home.

I frequently counsel IVF parents who are feeling distressed because they did not immediately feel profound love for their child. Parents expect the love to arrive as it does in the movies, immediately and without question.

I ask them how they felt about a good friend the day they met for the very first time. 'Were you immediately overwhelmed with regard for this person?' They usually shake their heads.

'What about your partner? Were you in love the second you first met?'

Again I usually see a shake of the head. They tell me that love and friendship both took time.

'Then love and regard will take time to come for your baby too,' I explain.

Giving birth is actually the first step in a long process of getting to know the baby and the baby getting to know his parents. He has been inside his mother's womb, giving him the chance to become familiar with her voice, her movements and her daily rituals of life. The mother gets to know all about the baby's movement patterns and perhaps his occasional bouts of hiccups. This does not constitute a rich and full human relationship, merely the very beginning of one.

Relationships are created between two people bound together by knowledge of each other. This knowledge takes time to develop in any new relationship, including that of mum and baby and of dad and baby. Thus birth is just the very beginning of a long journey of getting to know each other. No mum and dad can therefore expect to understand a new baby's cries, facial expressions or habits. Getting to know each other, and how to respond appropriately to your baby will take time.

As new parents of an IVF-conceived baby, you will probably feel many different emotions wash over you during the first one or two days after the birth. These feelings will come, sometimes intensely, and often depart just as quickly. You will probably feel shock that all you have been through has produced a real live baby. You may feel a tremendous sense of responsibility to care and provide for your child. You will also feel anxious to protect this precious baby and it may be hard to shut out the nagging worries that fill your head at times such as 'Is he healthy? Is there any issue

I should know about? What if ...?'

The best way to address these worries is by accepting they are part of parenting through IVF and ensuring you both talk to the doctor who examines your baby to hear that all is well. Also make sure you see the results of the Guthrie test, which is performed on all newborns by a heel prick and collection of a tiny drop of blood on the second day after birth. This test examines risk factors for more than thirty genetic and metabolic disorders and a healthy 'pass' is of great reassurance to parents.

You may be worried that you are not up to the task of parenting, despite the months and years of wanting a baby. These feelings are entirely normal, very common and have absolutely no bearing on how you will ultimately parent.

Your job in the first days is to simply acknowledge the variety of feelings you experience, perhaps talk about them with your partner, and watch as they go again.

Mothers may go through many bouts of tears in the first day or two. Part of this involves the normal hormonal adjustment, often termed the 'baby blues'. This is not post-natal depression, nor does it indicate you are likely to suffer from this. It is a normal process of emotional expression that may well serve the purpose of helping you psychologically come to terms with pregnancy, birth and the adjustment to parental responsibility. The first days are actually a useful time to have this reaction because it draws a partner, together with family and professionals, around you to offer assistance at the time you most need it. Tears really do serve an important function, so do not be afraid of shedding them.

You may both find it helpful to 'debrief': talk over every stage of the birth over the coming days and weeks. Women, particularly, need to discuss a big event a number of times. This is not usually a man's method and if, as the male partner coping after birth, you find your partner needs to talk, try to let her discuss her concerns. This is not a sign of anything amiss but a healthy psychological process at work.

If either of you find it too upsetting to talk about the birth, this may be a sign you are a little stuck in the process of achieving peace of mind over what happened on the day of the birth. It is important not to overreact to birth distress, but also not to pretend it did not happen and therefore your feelings are wrong. If either partner feels upset, talk to your doctor, midwife or nurse and be guided by their advice. Most of this distress goes away after a few weeks, but may need a little support in doing so. If you feel too distressed to focus on taking your baby home, make this known to staff. This does not mean you are not going to be a great parent (you will be). It simply means you need to resolve one or two issues before you begin preparations to start your life as a family at home.

For parents of multiple babies, the first few days in hospital can be an overwhelming experience. With two or more babies, you will be receiving more than the usual attention from everyone you meet. Most parents of multiples say they felt quite numb in the first few days; it is hard to take in the presence of the babies after the worry of the pregnancy and birth. Hospital can also be a very busy time getting to know the babies and establishing patterns of feeding.

The mother of twins told me, 'Having the babies was a busy time and I was overwhelmed with lack of sleep and dealing with two at once.' If this is your experience, do not be afraid to ask midwives for help and think about how friends and relatives can also assist you, perhaps by coming to the hospital to look after the babies while you enjoy a shower. The most important point to remember is to show your emotions, not to hide them. Some parents can be so focused on 'holding things together' that no one realises they are not coping. As parents of multiples, you are entitled to ask for more help.

6

Early Days

*I had wanted babies so desperately and for so long that I really
didn't know why I wasn't on cloud nine.*

The twins 'are our reward for years of infertility, and for having to go
through the emotional roller coaster that is IVF,' an IVF mother said.

Getting ready to leave hospital often brings moments of mixed emotions
for very new parents. Elation at finally being able to be a normal family is
blended with sheer panic at the responsibility of caring for this tiny life.
Couples are no longer surrounded by professionals providing help.

As brand-new IVF parents, the baby will seem so precious and vulnerable. Now is the time to use the survival guide you made before you went
into hospital.

Accept any offers of help. Many people do not enjoy relying on outside
help and the father may feel it is his role to look after his new family. But
have a relative or friend buy essential food for you both, for a few days
after you return home, and friends may bring over home-cooked meals
you can reheat. The first few evenings out of hospital may be the most
unsettled for a newborn and a nutritious dinner you do not have to cook
yourselves can nurture your tired soul.

It may not be a good idea to be all alone right after leaving hospital, but the opposite, a stampede of relatives and friends, rarely works either. You will both be tired from the events of the past days, possibly emotional and hardly sociable, so companionship needs to come in the form of a discreet friend or relative who can help without expecting anything in return. Save the large parties of visitors for a few weeks while you adjust to being parents.

First-night nerves

In my experience, the parents' first night home with an IVF-conceived newborn baby seems either particularly wonderful or fairly horrific; rarely is there a middle ground. This probably has more to do with the parents' expectations than with what actually happens during this momentous night. Therefore, try to be realistic.

Most newborn babies wake for feeding every three to four hours throughout the night and may take up to forty minutes or even an hour to feed each time. Newborns who sleep through the night are so rare as to be virtually unheard of. Most new parents respond more slowly to newborns than to older babies because their 'baby senses' require practise to become finely tuned. Each time you settle down after feeding, set an alarm clock for four hours to ensure you can rest without worrying about not hearing the baby cry.

Newborns will cry at night and may not be soothed straight away, no matter what wonderful technique you use. This does not relate to the quality of your parenting skills.

Around 3 to 5 am is the most difficult time for a human to be awake, so do not expect to enjoy this feed at all. This does not make you a bad parent.

If you are breastfeeding, you will very likely experience some nipple soreness. This has nothing to do with your technique and everything to do with the fact that it takes a few weeks for nipples to become used to the job.

Tuck your baby loosely into her cot or bassinet and position her close to you if at all possible: newborns are programmed to feel safe and therefore sleepy with the audible rhythm of their parents' breathing. When you feed during the night, keep the lights dim, avoid talking to your baby and avoid eye contact too: all of these techniques help her learn that night-time is for sleeping. Above all, try not to worry about tomorrow, next week or even next month and feel proud of what you have both achieved. This is even more important if you are the fragile parents of twins or triplets.

Are babies helpless?

Beginning life as a family involves getting to know one another. Some new parents look at me aghast when I say this, wondering how they can get to know a helpless infant. Be aware that each newborn has many skills designed to help him form a relationship with his parents so he can grow and thrive. Knowing these skills helps parents feel the baby's fragility just a little less.

The American paediatrician Berry Brazelton is renowned for his novel approach to the assessment of newborn skills. His research has revealed a little of what newborn babies are capable of and how they communicate with us.[1] His work shows that the months of pregnancy have led to a baby with prior experiences from inside the womb and a wonderful array of skills to cope with the world. Brazelton stresses that understanding an individual newborn's behaviour gives parents a much clearer understanding of what will help him. There is nothing worse than to be faced with a clearly distressed newborn yet have no idea what the cause of the distress could be.

There are four important patterns of behaviour to note when forming a bond with your baby.

The ability to mimic

Newborns may open and close their mouths in response to a parent talking to them closely. They can focus to a degree on a face and are primed to be sociable, so have time with your baby close to you where you can see each other's faces. Be aware of your baby beginning to look away when she has had enough of being sociable.

Difficulty coping with stimulation

If your baby constantly looks away from light or noise or startles at even a muffled noise, his nervous system may be especially sensitive. This is particularly true for babies born even a little prematurely. To help, try to reduce noise around your newborn, talk quietly to him, hold him firmly and keep him wrapped up so he feels safe until his nervous system matures a little.

Shutting out light and noise

Some newborns struggle to shut out light and noise while they sleep. Others hear a loud vacuum cleaner, the drill from renovations next door and a car whizzing by and fall asleep! If you have a newborn that wakes very regularly, have her bassinet in a dim room, perhaps with dark curtains at the windows. Play lullabies softly while she sleeps to help avoid other noises outside startling her. Avoid going in to the room to check on her regularly and disturbing her; use a baby monitor instead.

Born settlers

Some babies can be placed in a bassinet and will be able to fall asleep without help. Many others need their parents to soothe them before they can fall asleep. To identify your baby's type, place him in his bassinet when he is fussing after being fed and after a little waking time. Pat him gently, softly tell him it is time to sleep and leave him. It is fine to leave a baby to fuss intermittently, but not one who is clearly distressed and crying. The secret of this technique is learning to distinguish between fussing and real distress: 'fussing' is when your baby makes intermittent, short cries, talks to himself or makes noises designed to say, 'Are you there, Mum and Dad?'; 'distress' is when your baby cries continuously and the volume increases as time goes by. If your baby cannot settle and cries, go to him and gently pat him. Continue this routine for ten minutes. Move on to rocking him if his distress does not lessen. By three months of age, most babies are easily able to learn to settle themselves with this habitual pattern of settling.

Feeding

Issues over infant feeding can loom large for IVF families. Research reported in the *Handbook of Parenting*[1] reveal that IVF mothers report lowered self-esteem and confidence in parenting skills as compared to non-IVF mothers and this can impact upon the success of breastfeeding. Mothers often believe they are not producing enough milk to help their babies to thrive and may turn to bottle-feeding to supplement breast milk. There may be a link between mothers feeling their bodies cannot do the job of mothering after failing to get pregnant naturally and these mothers believing they cannot breastfeed adequately.

It is well worth investing time and energy in developing confidence about breastfeeding. Not only does it give babies a nutritional advantage, it also promotes a close bond between the baby and mother, who will feel more confident in her mothering.

As a new IVF parent, do not be afraid to call for help if breastfeeding is a struggle. Many new mothers find it tough to get breastfeeding well established: perhaps mastitis arises, latching on may be quite painful in the first few weeks, and a woman who is woken four times in a night to feed her baby may long for a rest. Try to appreciate that these problems are short-term and can be overcome as long as you are offered good support. Talk to your midwife, family doctor or local baby clinic if you do not feel confident about breastfeeding.

Coping

All parents of newborn babies feel they cannot cope sometimes. Even highly trained executives who run large companies, early childhood teachers used to large numbers of young children and doctors with medical know-how feel overwhelmed at times with a newborn. Those feelings will not last and they do not define parenting.

As the parent of a baby or babies conceived through IVF, research shows you are more likely to feel stress than parents who have conceived naturally. Some stress is good: it heightens your senses, gives you energy to cope and focuses your mind on the task at hand.

Too much stress, however, has a negative effect. Acute stress that is not relieved leads to the body maintaining 'fight or flight' responses as a means of survival. This state also produces poor memory and concentration, reduced food digestion and cell repair in the body and poor quality of sleep. Too much stress plays havoc with the mind and body and can lower your immune system.

Good stress management is therefore essential. There are seven stress reducers to help you stay sane in the first few weeks:

Sleep

Sleep deprivation is a form of torture, and a very effective one too. Sleep robs you of energy, pleasure and problem-solving skills. You will be sleep-deprived at times with a newborn, but you can reduce the damage done by a large sleep deficit by planning to catch up at every opportunity. Take it in turns to sleep in on days when the working partner is not at work. Try expressing milk if you are breastfeeding to allow your partner to do one feed each night. Try to take a nap during the day when the baby is asleep. If you have other children to care for, ask a friend or relative to take over for an hour every other day to allow you to have a rest. If you find it hard to get back to sleep after being woken during the night, use the Sanskrit chant. Remember your driving skills deteriorate when you are sleep-deprived, so take a cab to work, ask a friend to drive you to the shops or get what you need online and stay safely at home.

Food

Food is not just for energy; it is also a wonderful mood enhancer if you eat wisely. Now, in the middle of caring for a newborn, food has never been more important. You do not need to spend much time preparing meals for them to be valuable. Cereals made with oats are fantastic for energy. Wholemeal sandwiches filled with cold chicken, tuna fish, tinned salmon and salad also give a great boost to both body and mind. Fresh fruit is refreshing. Drink plenty of water as dehydration can add to exhaustion, and avoid too much caffeine, which gives you an instant 'up' only to be followed by a much lower 'down'.

Caring for yourself

A four-minute shower, a ten-minute facial, a chance to read the headlines in the newspaper and a snack enjoyed without trying to feed the baby at the same time are all quick but important ways to care for yourselves in the early days. Treasured small moments of time to think of 'you' ward off extreme stress. Perhaps you can ask each other for time to have a treat during the day. Ensure you thank your partner for this help.

Relationship dos

The fatigue and worry of the first weeks can easily lead to friction between partners. The solution is two-fold: firstly, accept there will be more arguments but that this is only temporary; secondly, try to always treat your partner with respect, no matter what is happening. At times of stress, it is easy to forget 'please' and 'thank you', but words are very powerful and can make someone feel much more positive. Also avoid criticising; you will both develop a different relationship with your baby and will not care for him in exactly the same way. This will not harm your baby, and in fact gives him a greater experience of the world.

Mild exercise

Exercise is one of the best anti-stress measures, for the simple reason that it reverses all the effects stress has on the body. Once you have taken a walk, fewer stress hormones will be circulating around your body, making you feel more relaxed and also less tired. Try to go for a ten-minute walk each day — make this twice a day if you possibly can. If you are very nervous about taking the baby out, something that may well be the case early on, ask your partner to do the caring just for a short while.

Asking for help

At times stressed parents can become very introverted, believing only they can solve the problems they face. I have also found that parents coming to terms with the safe arrival of a longed-for IVF-conceived baby can feel that only they must do the caring because no one else appreciates how precious she is. Both patterns of thought lead to acute stress in the early days, but there are alternative scenarios. As far as problem-solving goes, two heads are much better than one. If there is some issue to resolve in your lives as new parents — perhaps feeding is difficult, settling is not going well or you fear you are slipping into bad parenting habits — ask for assistance, from your partner or others around you. There is no pressure to accept the advice, but often talking with others about your difficulty can bring a new perspective. The supports you noted on your survival plan — a breastfeeding association, a counsellor you have used, your baby clinic and a parenting hotline — can all help you find solutions to your difficulties while making you feel less isolated and better supported during this time.

If you don't trust others with your precious child, be assured this is normal. However, it is in your own best interests to gradually learn to trust a select few people. First, choose the person you feel safest with, perhaps your own mother or a close friend. Begin by asking for very small amounts of help: perhaps your helper can hold the baby for a minute while you warm milk or change his bedding. Give clear instructions as to what you want, to ensure you feel safe and the helper knows what to do. Once you have gradually mastered coping with some help, graduate to bigger 'asks', such as leaving the baby with your chosen carer for ten minutes so you can shower or have a brief walk. The more you trust in a safe way, the easier you will find the process of getting the help you need.

If you or your partner finds it impossible to trust anyone due to your anxiety being too great, seek counselling, especially if one partner feels he or she cannot trust the other. At this stage, your fears can be addressed by simple-to-learn psychological techniques that will prevent you from having to 'go it alone' in parenting.

Time for bonding for both of you

As your relationship with your baby deepens, so you will be better able to interpret his signals and more able to feel empathy for his needs, even at 2 am. This parent-baby bond is the 'pull' that keeps a parent coming back to the child no matter how tough the relationship is. The bond does require time to grow and that means you and your baby spending time together, enjoying each other and discovering how you fit together.

A mother often begins to feel this bond grow as breastfeeding settles and she is able to comfort her baby most of the time. The bond rarely appears instantly, and feeling guilty that you have not yet 'fallen in love' with your baby can get in the way of a bond forming. Give the relationship time. Every day take time to study the baby's face, allow her to study yours and make faces to watch her try to imitate you. Quiet study of each other is a wonderful way to strengthen your bond. Also read the Dr Seuss books to your baby, who will love the sound of your voice and the rhythm of the words.

As a brand-new father, you also need time to bond with your baby. If you need to return to work quickly, this bonding can take longer and may generate some frustration as your partner moves further ahead in her understanding. She may also feel the need to show you 'what to do'. Try not to react negatively to this and instead reassure her that you are enjoying time with your child as she is enjoying time with you.

A 2006 survey found that 84 per cent of new mothers believe their partners fail to bond with their newborns because of work commitments.[2] When conception has been through IVF, the father may have additional fears over his competence and the baby's vulnerability which keep him even further away emotionally. For the sake of your baby, your partner and your own self-esteem as a father, closing this gap is essential. Every dad needs to have his own rituals with his newborn. It will take time for you to develop your own ways of interacting with your baby. Some suggestions to build this precious bond include: taking a 10 or 11 pm feed using expressed milk in a bottle, giving the baby a bath each evening, and ten minutes of talking quietly to the child or reading a story.

If, as a mother, you feel your partner is less competent than you are, try not to point this out but identify tasks he does really well and praise him for this. Help him out quietly if he asks for assistance, but also recognise that he will develop his own ways of caring for his child as time passes.

Goals for weeks one to six

The first six weeks of caring for a tiny baby, particularly a first child, are exhausting and fairly stressful. For parents who have brought home a newborn conceived following IVF, the stresses of this time may well be exaggerated. As new IVF parents, it will help you to have a focus for your efforts in the early weeks of parenting.

Avoid isolation

Anyone who has gone through a somewhat abnormal event will feel some isolation. If you have had a serious illness, a traffic accident or been involved in a natural disaster, at times you will feel 'different' and isolated from people who have not experienced trauma as you have. As IVF parents, you will, like parents of premature babies, often feel different and you can easily feel isolated, believing no one understands your experiences.

One of the most valuable ways to reduce this isolation is to talk with other parents who have successfully conceived and given birth after IVF treatment. In an instant, you move from feeling isolated to feeling understood and not at all alone. Other IVF parents talk your language. You may have already met other parents while going through IVF, but many couples say they rarely keep in touch as the stress and fear of failure, inherent in the process, makes it hard to talk to other couples who are going through those same difficulties. But in the early days of parenting, a support group becomes an important option.

The easiest method of getting in contact with other IVF parents is through the national infertility organisation, which operates a special group for IVF parents who are able to email, phone or meet each other (see Useful Contacts, page 201). Another source of potential understanding can come from other parents who may have suffered infertility, perhaps those who have used infertility drug therapy to conceive. Your local baby clinic may be able to put you in touch with such parents; it will also assign you to a group of mothers who have all given birth at a similar time, a way of providing support and understanding — and playmates for the babies. New mothers describe these groups as 'life-savers'.

For those who have IVF-conceived babies, mothers' groups can be a wonderful way to share new mothering, but they can have tough moments. One woman told me that she was fine until one of the other mothers said breezily, 'I got pregnant the first time of trying. Am I worried about going for a second close to this one? No, I most certainly am not!' Despite such problems, these groups provide very important social opportunities. Studies of IVF parents reveal that overall these parents use less social support, a fact that can lead to greater stress and a reduced ability to cope with the demands of parenting. Mothers' groups can be one way to address this isolation and it is worth coping with the feelings of being different that may come from time to time.

Prioritise

One of the best techniques to master is the ability to prioritise. Without developing this skill, it is easy for new parents to feel overwhelmed with the sheer number of tasks that remain undone. No one anticipates just how much time a tiny baby occupies in the day. You need to be calm in order to plan sensibly. One method is to set aside five minutes in the morning to plan the day ahead together, as a couple, perhaps while you are feeding your baby. Take a few deep breaths before you start, to relax and get the brain working. Make a list of everything that is essential today, such as making bottles, fixing a pile of washing, bathing the baby and perhaps ordering the shopping. Next, allocate who will do this so you both know what you need to achieve. Perhaps choose one extra task such as vacuuming that you would like to get done and add this as a 'wish item'. Try to avoid fretting if your extra task remains undone at the day's end; simply add it to the next day's list. Try to think only of today rather than worrying about all that you have to do tomorrow or next week. Any stress you are already feeling becomes multiplied several thousand times if you begin to look too far ahead.

SIDS precautions

With the anxiety that follows the birth of a much longed-for baby, fears over SIDS (sudden infant death syndrome) loom large for most parents. The best method of allaying the worst of those fears is to be fully informed of the risks and act to protect your baby.

The known risk factors are:

- *Sleeping on the tummy or side*. If babies sleep on their backs, their risk of SIDS is reduced by half. Make sure he always sleeps on his back. Once he can roll over, he will assume his own favoured method of sleeping.
- *Smoking in the family*, particularly that of the mother. Parents should not smoke, particularly in your baby's first year of life. The ideal is never to smoke.

- *Excess clothing or wrapping.* Young babies are not able to throw off covers if they get too hot. Make sure the baby is wrapped only in a very light cotton wrap. Use bedding consistent with the temperature in the room; for example, a warm twenty-four degrees may warrant only a cotton vest and the wrap. Check the baby's forehead to see how warm he feels if there are concerns.

- *Avoid bed sharing.* Instead, have a baby in a cot or bassinet next to your bed. This way, the baby has all the benefits of being close to his parents without the risk of overheating or being covered by blankets.

Other factors that may help include: breastfeeding, which may offer some protection but as yet there is no conclusive proof and no reason for parents who bottle-feed to worry; the use of a dummy, which may help to keep airways open more easily although, again, there is no conclusive proof, and treating respiratory illnesses because SIDS may have a viral link.

Involving grandparents

From an emotional perspective, IVF remains in its infancy and parents' needs are often not met, never mind those of grandparents. A lack of understanding and support for grandparents can lead to friction between parents and grandparents once the baby is home. Grandparents are likely to feel stress resulting from infertility and IVF treatment, even though they may not live near their son or daughter, or even in the same country. It is highly distressing for grandparents to see their child, no matter an adult one, grieving over the inability to conceive naturally and having to endure the difficult components of IVF treatment. They may cope in many ways, some positive and others that can even hurt the new family. I have witnessed grandparents who simply could not get enough information about what was happening and drove the IVF parents crazy with incessant phone calls. These calls began from the time the couple started trying to have a baby right through until after the birth. Other grandparents have been so fearful over this 'new' technology that they stay away and change the subject from babies to avoid having to confront their fears.

But grandparents can be wonderfully supportive, at times smothering, at others mildly aggressive, and sometimes quietly happy. My own view is that their reactions are generally very hard to predict.

We all have ideas about how our parents will support us when we have our own children. These expectations come from many different experiences: the kind of support our parents received from their parents; the help parents gave to another sibling, witnessing how much support friends with babies got from their parents, and inevitably from the media. Most of the time, what we expect is not quite what we get and this can be very disappointing to struggling new parents.

The key to managing the grandparent relationship is to keep your expectations realistic and to make sure positive input from the grandparents is highlighted and praised. Expectations that a set of grandparents will care for your baby for long periods while you work may not be realistic as many older people wish to enjoy a quieter life and find childcare very demanding. Older grandparents, especially, will be limited in any care they can handle and you must ensure they are able to care for a baby safely. If their own health is poor, child-minding is perhaps best offered to another family member, friend or professional carer.

Another common expectation is that these new grandparents will be able and willing to treat the baby as her parents wish. Many older people interact with children in a different way: they may seem blunt or even harsh at times, reflecting the styles of parenting of the mid-twentieth century. They may not wish to, or even be able to, interact in the way you would wish. If you are concerned about their style of interaction with a grandchild, handle this by role modelling careful parenting yourselves and minimise the time your child has alone with her grandparent.

Other expectations that women often have about their own mothers is that they will be willing and empathic listeners. As a brand-new mother of an IVF baby, there will be many frustrations and fears over early parenting that you may wish to talk over with your mother and seek reassurance and comfort about. However, some grandmothers find it very hard to listen to their daughters expressing unhappiness, particularly when the difficulties of infertility have turned to the delight of a healthy baby. Mothers may be brisk and unsympathetic with a daughter, they may exert pressure on her to speak only of the delights of parenting and they may even criticise her for voicing unhappiness. The solution is to try to accept your mother may not necessarily be your most empathic listener and to find another family member or close friend to fill that role.

Be assured, praising your parents for their positive input into your new family does help, although it may take time to practise the technique. The point about praise is that it makes a person much more likely to repeat the behaviour that earned the praise. If your father is able to put his arm around you and say, 'Well done', take the time to ensure he knows how much this means to you. If grandparents are able to watch the baby even for thirty minutes, let them know it made an important difference.

Just as parents need time to form a relationship with their baby, so grandparents need to take the time to form a bond with their grandchild, and to adjust their relationship with the child's mother and father now they are parents. Relationships usually become much less strained as time goes by.

The six-week check

The six-week medical check is an important marker for new parents. Not only is it time for the mother and baby to be medically assessed, it is also a good time to reflect on the last six weeks as a couple, to talk about the highs and lows of new parenting and to ascertain if there are any potentially serious issues that need to be dealt with. It is useful for both parents to attend the six-week check if possible, so they can raise any points they are concerned about.

Six weeks generally marks the time when the mother should be feeling more like herself physically. After a vaginal delivery, stitches will have been taken out and tears should have healed quite well. A caesarean section scar should be healing and discomfort much reduced. She should be feeling less bruised and battered, losing weight and the initial trials of sore nipples during breastfeeding should be over. The check at the doctor's office or clinic is a good time to review how you are feeling, to be honest about any physical issues and to reflect on your emotional well-being.

It is also important to have the baby checked by a paediatrician at this stage. Many IVF pregnancies generate enormous concern for parents over the health of the baby and these concerns can continue unchecked after the birth. To address these concerns, and to prevent irrational fears building, a thorough check gives both parents the chance to raise any fears, to learn how their baby is doing and to have feedback on their parenting so far. Most of the time this is an opportunity for a doctor to confirm to parents that their baby is healthy, happy and progressing entirely normally — feedback that is essential after infertility and IVF experiences. Even if a concern is noted, you can assess what to do and be reassured as to how much notice should be given to the issue rather than face the uncertainty of not knowing.

As a new father, the six-week check also marks a time to assess how you are faring. Both your female partner and your baby need you to cope and it is important to be honest about how you are managing your many demands. If you are back at work, review how the balance of home and work is faring and how much sleep you are getting. If you are feeling overwhelmed, this is a good time for both of you to discuss options, such as slightly reduced working hours, a different and less demanding area of responsibility or the possibility of taking long-service leave or unpaid holiday. These short-term measures can ease stress for the whole family.

Finally, this is the time to evaluate how feeding and settling are working for your baby. Both are intrinsically linked: the safest and happiest state a baby can be in is when he is well fed. Both breast- and bottle-feeding take time to establish for a newborn; by six weeks, however, feeding should be more routine and of less concern. If this is not the case — perhaps breast-feeding is still painful, mastitis has been an issue, the baby has been prone to fussy feeding or vomiting feeds, or a mixed breast/bottle baby is experiencing confusion — now is the time to seek help.

Minor breastfeeding concerns can be addressed to the breastfeeding counsellor. Major feeding and settling concerns should be taken first to your doctor to rule out medical conditions and then to a family care unit. Your family doctor can give you a referral.

Family care centres have facilities for parents and babies to stay from one day to one week. Centres are staffed by specialist nurses and may also have social workers and counsellors for parents who require psychological support. The benefits of such support are substantial for most families: a chance to feel less alone, advice on breast- and bottle-feeding, help with settling restless babies and assistance in establishing daily routines. This may also be the chance for the couple to talk to a counsellor about any relationship issues that have arisen.

Goals for weeks seven to twelve

Settling

The frustrations of the early days usually give way to a more organised pattern of settling by seven weeks. Parents may still be feeding or rocking their baby to sleep at the end of each awake period, but now they can begin to start teaching their baby to settle herself.

For your IVF baby, settling herself to sleep unaided is an important developmental milestone. This is the baby's first gain of independence, one that will give her feelings of safety and security, as well as increased self-esteem. As parents anxious to do your best, you may fear this means leaving her to cry. This is not the case; there are safe ways to teach your baby to settle without having to resort to her crying for long periods.

Settling is an art for your baby to learn over a week or two. You can look out for signs that she is ready to self-settle by putting her in her cot when normally she would be sleepy. Leave her with a mobile or other object of interest nearby, perhaps while you take an evening shower. The key to this technique is that you leave your baby if she is fussing, making discontinuous noises. Only if she begins to cry continuously do you go to her. Initially, she may get tired of being alone and eventually need settling in her normal way. After a few weeks, you can increase the time she spends alone trying to settle herself, going in to soothe her if she cries but leaving again when she is settled. Eventually, you will walk in one day to find her sound asleep.

Your baby may have occasions of being over-tired and fretful even after she has learned self-soothing. Avoid the temptation to rock her to sleep unless she is unwell, and instead return to going in to her, patting or talking to her and leaving again when she is calm. This may take five or even ten trips but it is well worth the effort as your baby gets older.

The baby's settling can reflect the parents' state of mind in the early weeks. I often find that parents ask for help because she simply will not settle and they are finding it hard to settle themselves. The baby picks up parental anxiety: if you are both sleeping poorly outside of waking to give feeds, often your baby will too.

If this sounds like your family, you are not alone or abnormal. Plenty of families feel anxious and unsettled with a new baby, and those using IVF tend to feel the unease even more. Please contact your family doctor for a referral to a parenting centre or a specialist infant counsellor who can help both you and your baby to settle into your new relationships.

Developmental milestones

From seven weeks, your baby's smiles become more frequent and have more purpose. He can make small noises as you talk to him, the very beginning of his conversational ability. Start by talking to him, waiting for his reaction and again taking up the conversation. He can learn that social communication is all about both speaking and listening.

He is able to focus on objects of interest: faces further away from him and objects such as mobiles hung over his change table or cot. He can lift his head a little and may enjoy lying on the floor for short periods, on a soft play mat. He is becoming more aware of his own body so play gently with his hands and toes.

Being a good parent

Anxious parents rarely take the time to consider what they are doing right, often focusing instead on their perceived shortcomings. The latter part of the first three months after the baby is born is a wonderful time to focus on your achievements.

I ask parents to tell me what evidence they have that they are good parents. Many falter, feeling there is none. I then highlight the hugely important fact that a baby gaining weight is a sure sign that the parents are getting it right. A baby beginning to mimic facial expressions and smiling is another sure sign of parental success. Babies without tender loving care fail to thrive, they rarely put on weight and they fail to meet developmental milestones. We are creatures who need to be nurtured in order to survive and thrive. Every time your baby is weighed, give yourselves a mental pat on the back. Each time your baby smiles, congratulate yourselves on a job very well done. You are a good parent.

Special babies

Some babies are born needing extra care to survive and thrive. If this is your experience, both of you as parents will also need extra help and support to do your critically important job.

Premature and low-birthweight babies

Babies born through IVF, particularly multiples, tend to be born earlier and to weigh less than naturally conceived babies. Some IVF babies will need very special care at first. Both premature babies (born before thirty-seven weeks) and full-term low-birthweight babies are likely to spend longer in hospital than term babies within the usual weight range. This time in hospital after the mother has gone home can be extremely worrying for parents. 'My surviving son spent five weeks in special care, away from me. I was a part-time mum and the nurses knew more about how to care for my son than I did,' one mother of twins said.

Intensive care and special care units for newborns are high-pressure places for parents. Simply passing the sign directing visitors to the unit can fill them with dread. That said, parents can be the very best support possible for their baby if they consider adopting the following coping techniques:

- *Ask for information.* Doctors are very realistic about babies' conditions and that allows parents to understand and face the issues their baby is facing. However, it is often the case that stressed parents cannot take in or even remember what is said at the first hearing. Do not be afraid to ask for information again, even if you feel you may be wasting a doctor's precious time. Your baby needs you to be fully informed about his care.

- *Explore the baby's equipment.* The equipment around your baby can look frightening. If your baby is monitored, machines may be sounding alarms frequently, something that sends many parents into absolute panic. Ask the nurse caring for your baby to explain in simple terms what these machines are doing and which common alarms going off do not require you to panic.

- *Find routines for each day.* When my premature baby was in hospital over a decade ago, I comforted myself with a daily routine, which was a structure to hold on to when there was little else that was stable in life. Every day I woke at 7 am, expressed milk, went into the hospital and gave my son his 9 am bottle-feed of expressed milk (breastfeeding was too exhausting for him at first). This was a feed that I took great pleasure in providing for him. Then it was an hour of stroking him when he was undergoing phototherapy due to jaundice and had to remain in the incubator, and then later it was a cuddle. Around eleven, I would head off for a tea break to ensure I had the energy to continue the milk supply. Then it was back for the noon feed, more expressing, more talking to my baby and finally about half-past four home to my older son. In the evening after my eldest went to bed, it was a call to the hospital, more expressing, and a diary entry covering progress each day, followed by as much sleep as I could manage.

- *Learn baby massage.* The amazing Touch Research Institute in Florida, run by psychologist Dr Tiffany Field, has studied the benefits of massage for premature and low-birthweight babies for more than a decade. Their results show that infant massage can increase weight gain, organise behaviour and reduce the baby's stress levels. Massage also gives parents, who feel helpless in the hospital, the chance to perform a vital function for their babies, forming a special bond that benefits all. See Useful Contacts, page 201, for details of how to find a baby massage instructor.

- *Avoid catastrophising.* Most premature parents I have worked with, mothers especially, react to the drama of early birth by expecting everything to go wrong afterwards. They interpret a small setback, perhaps a temporary need for increased oxygen, as the end of the world. Several days of such catastrophising exhausts every ounce of energy they have. You need to preserve energy, and your sanity, by trying to view each event as just another small part of your baby's development. Setbacks come and go but rarely are they anything more than temporary. Try to acknowledge that setbacks are a hard, but very normal, part of IVF and try not to anticipate trouble if you are not sure it will really happen.

Bringing your baby home

Babies born prematurely tend to be more sensitive and more fretful in their early months compared with term babies. They cry more too. It is important to understand your baby crying a great deal is not about your standards of care but her own nervous system, which is very immature.

Bringing a premature baby home is a stressful experience and parents are wise to get as much help as they possibly can. Your baby will need calm, quiet handling for some time. Wrapping firmly is important because premature babies find it hard to still their movements at times and they can easily repeatedly disturb their own sleep. Talking gently to the baby will help her to recognise your voice and face. Avoiding too many people coming to visit at one time also helps and early outings should be kept to quiet walks. Premature babies are particularly averse to highly stimulating, busy shopping malls, so if you need to shop, try to do so early in the morning or online.

Once you have your baby home, you may find you feel very emotional. While the baby is in hospital, most parents feel quite numb and devoid of feelings. This can change quite dramatically once your baby is safe and thriving at home. It is very normal for the mother to first suffer a period of anxiety and tearfulness and later for dad to have a period of irritability. If this does not fade after two or three weeks, contact the social workers at the hospital where your baby was born to obtain a referral to a counselling professional.

A special mention must be made for parents of babies born very prematurely. As twenty-eight weeks has always been regarded as the time when survival is possible, babies under this age face a greater fight for life. Going into labour very prematurely is a terrifying experience, as is sitting by an intensive care cot, often for many weeks. Australia has adopted guidelines designed to help both doctors and parents make decisions about how to treat very premature infants. They recommend no resuscitation of babies born under twenty-three weeks' gestation. At twenty-three and twenty-four weeks, treatment may be offered, depending on the baby's condition and parents' wishes. Babies born at twenty-five to twenty-eight weeks are usually treated, because the odds of survival are much greater.

Any parent who goes through a very premature birth can benefit a great deal from counselling, no matter what the outcome is for their baby. These parents are very traumatised by their experiences and can find it hard to deal with normal life. Counselling can help to support them in the early weeks, helping them to adopt healthy coping strategies. And you can arrange to talk to the social workers at the hospital where your delivery took place if you find yourselves suffering anxiety once your baby is at home. Social workers will be able to provide you with a suitable contact to obtain counselling.

Multiple babies

Multiples are definitely more stressful to parents than single babies for a number of reasons. And recent studies have shown that for parents of twins conceived through IVF, parenting is more stressful than for parents of twins conceived without treatment. However, there is no evidence that babies conceived through IVF are harder to care for — rather, it is likely that stress in parenting for IVF parents follows on from stress throughout IVF treatment and the pregnancy.

Multiples pose health issues and logistical problems for parents. Health-wise, multiples face a higher risk of prematurity and/or abnormality and illness. The more babies there are, the greater the risk of health problems. Parents of multiples born prematurely will need to use the strategies out-lined above.

Homecoming for multiple babies may well be a staggered affair, with the heaviest of the babies released from hospital first. If this does happen, parents get a chance to get used to caring for one or perhaps two babies before the smallest arrives. As with all babies born before thirty-seven weeks, premature multiples may be particularly sensitive. So having a quiet house, wrapping the babies firmly, and close and quiet face-to-face contact will work well. Research seems to show that keeping the babies close together, with skin-on-skin contact as they were in the womb, is also a comfort for them.

Parents of multiples always say routine and order is what kept them sane during the first year. Routine means trying to get the babies' sleeping patterns into sync by waking all when one wakes for a feed or staggering wake up and feeding times so one baby is fed and enjoying awake time when the other wakes. You may choose to breastfeed. You can consider the option of expressing milk as well to allow others to help, or if you have twins, you may wish to talk to a lactation consultant about the positions for breastfeeding both babies at the same time. Breastfeeding can take longer to establish for multiples, so try not to become frustrated in the early days. 'I had a hard time breastfeeding and I really wanted to because I knew it was so good for them. Once I had settled into the breastfeeding and had got used to the lack of sleep, I started to enjoy my babies more and feel more capable,' a mother of boy/girl twins said. Some parents of multiples find a mixture of breast milk and formula works for them: remember your health and sanity as a parent is as important as the way your babies are fed, and there are many formula-fed babies who grow up to be athletes, highly intelligent academics and shrewd business people.

Routines for multiple babies work best if you have regular help, such as a grandparent coming at 5 pm each day to bathe the babies while you organise a meal. As multiple parents, you may also wish to consider hiring a student, who arrives at 4 pm each day when the babies are at their most demanding and two pairs of hands are required. It is also helpful for your partner to arrive home at a regular time every evening to assist in getting the babies into bed.

Order for multiple parents is a useful concept. Order may mean employing strategies to organise bottles, dummies, clothes and toys. Psychological research has shown that multiples fare better if right from the outset they are treated as individuals with their own belongings. To achieve this, a colour-coding system is essential, one colour for each baby from homecoming and sewn or marked on every belonging.

Parents of multiples often express grief in the early months for being far too busy to really be close to any one of their babies. Feeding, settling, bathing, nappy changing and home management for two or more babies rarely gives time for them to engage in the relaxed interactions that parents of one baby often enjoy. I feel parents cope better with the early trials of parenting when strong bonds develop between parent and baby and so always encourage parents of multiples to try to have time alone with each baby, even if this is but ten minutes every other day. If you are offered help, having a helper cuddle one or more babies while you have relaxing, one-on-one time with one baby brings enormous benefits for you and your babies. Parents of multiples also need to know they do not always have to take all babies out wherever they go. Taking one baby out each time you go and leaving the other behind with your partner makes life easier and much more enjoyable on occasions.

Special needs babies

Babies with illnesses or disabilities are very special and so are their parents. Coming to terms with a baby who has special needs takes time and enormous amounts of energy, and it rarely happens before the family leaves the safety of hospital. The first months require a great deal of help and support from professionals, family and friends and some thinking about how to simplify the normal aspects of living.

Special needs babies may be under the care of paediatricians, specialist doctors, occupational therapists, physiotherapists, speech therapists, and so on. Organising appointments and keeping track of what each specialist requires to be done can be tricky.

Dad has a huge role to play in the early weeks, as he is often the most valuable planner and organiser whilst mum is chief nurturer. Dad can be of great help by organising a list of drugs to administer, hospital appointments to attend and exercises to do whilst keeping track of these on a daily basis. It is also highly useful to create a box file with test results, letters from doctors and referrals to ensure that no important information goes missing.

Sleep is a crucial part of finding acceptance of what has happened. The brain processes difficulties during sleep: sleep-deprived parents do not heal properly. The best help you can ask for at first is someone to care for the baby while you sleep.

Another crucial part of parenting special needs babies in the early weeks is avoiding isolation. Many parents feel guilt, shame or simply feel too overwhelmed, and cannot face family and friends. The isolation intensifies grief and anger, common components of the early days. Whatever you do, try to garner face-to-face support from at least a few trusted friends and close family members. You can also contact the hospital your baby attends for details of any local support groups or national support organisations you can join.

The early weeks will be less traumatic if you are able to form a strong bond with your baby. Strong connections form when both of you can study each other, you can hold your baby close in your arms, talk gently to him and notice how he responds to you. If you are unable to do this because of grief or intense feelings of other kinds, please contact your family doctor or the hospital social workers for a referral to a counselling professional.

7

Are We Good Enough?

The twins are our reward for years of infertility, and for having to go through the emotional roller coaster that is IVF.

From the slightly calmer three-month stage until a child reaches school, most IVF parents have their attention focused firmly on being good parents. This is normal. New parenting is the time you are most motivated to make changes in your lives to create happy families, and if you had unhappy times as children, the motivation can be particularly strong.

For parents whose babies arrived through IVF, 'good parenting' takes on a whole new meaning. There are two reasons for this. The first concerns the efforts put into achieving a pregnancy. Something couples have longed for, dreamed about and waited an eternity to have takes on a far greater significance than something that occurred easily. This is a fundamental trait: some of life's treasures are so important that humans are willing to sacrifice much to be able to have them, so achieving them make them highly prized. IVF couples thus feel their parenting must be of the highest quality, as though they need to earn the right to parent their child. The second reason is the belief that achieving something that has been so difficult must have made everyone consistently happy. I sense many parents who have an IVF baby feel that the arrival of their child should signal completion of their happiness and an end to any difficulties whatsoever. This can be the result of the bargaining that normally happens as a response to grief (see pages 11–12), when couples may think: 'If I can just achieve a family, I'll never ask for anything again, and my life will be complete.'

Both reasons mean parents are highly motivated to care for any children conceived through IVF and their levels of care are wonderfully high. I have never had to help IVF parents pay more attention to their babies, but on occasions mothers who had unplanned babies have needed to learn this.

The high standards IVF parents set themselves are not harmful to the child's development. Rather, it seems an agonising task for these parents to work out how good is 'good enough'. Frequently, parents tear themselves apart trying to be just a little better. This is accentuated even more if the child is likely to be the only one the couple will have. 'After all,' one mother said, 'we don't have the luxury of doing it better second time around.'

As the wise rabbi Harold Kushner described in his book *How Good Do We Have to Be?*, both parents and children may have unrealistic expectations about how the parent-child relationship will be. This sums up the struggle IVF parents have during their years of raising children. After IVF, the theme of 'are we good enough?' seems acutely burned into their brains, leaving little space for them to stop and simply enjoy parenting. It also prevents them from being able to admit that 'I don't need to be perfect.'

IVF parents, even more than other parents, need regular reality checks. They need to be helped to focus on what is normal, healthy and acceptable, rather than on what is wrong, deficient or not worthy of their miracle child. This reality check is something I help parents focus on regularly, offering them a chance to reflect on their parenting, their parents' parenting and their child's functioning. Such reflection centres on two main areas.

The pleasures of parenting

The most important piece of parenting advice I ever received when my children were small was that pleasure comes in small bursts, and it is to be welcomed and enjoyed whenever possible. Above all, parenting is hard and can be very frustrating at times. There are no days off, holidays or monetary bonuses, and rarely pats on the back from others. There will be times, I assure all parents, when they feel less than competent for the task at hand, and even occasions when they struggle to like their child's behaviour even as they love them completely. All these aspects of being a parent are entirely normal and a sign of being a very typical human being.

On the other hand, there are those moments, fleeting at first, of great contentment in being a real family and immense pleasure in holding a beautiful baby. These moments need to be savoured. I remember the first time I allowed my firstborn to fall asleep in my arms and refused to move him, so much was I enjoying the physical contact. It was bliss and I still remember the warmth of that love and the wonder I felt looking at his newly emerging curves. I fell in love at that point in a way that I had not been able to allow myself to do in the first two chaotic months. It was a revelation.

Later on, there was the joy of cuddling up with a sleepy boy after a busy day, and giving in to the demand of 'Just one more story, Mummy.' During these moments all the difficulties of parenting simply fell from my mind, the dirty dishes downstairs disappeared and the laundry flew away Mary Poppins-style. Then there was the first time my youngest said 'I love you Mummy' thirty minutes after a particularly brutal tantrum. And there was the first gift from preschool, a manically coloured scrap of paper that was 'Mum' in all her stick figure glory. These are the precious moments that all parents need to savour, IVF parents particularly.

Getting it wrong

Why is it so important to be wrong sometimes? In reality, perfect parents are dangerous parents. A child will eventually go off alone into the big, wide world where all manner of trials, disappointments and hurts are waiting. This does not mean she won't also experience joys, triumphs and happiness, but these will come and go. Life is tough at times for all of us.

As perfect parents, you cannot teach your children the valuable lessons of what to do when you mess up. Your cannot demonstrate what to do when someone else messes up and, even more importantly, what to do when you just can't find a way through. An adult, especially a parent, getting it wrong is the way that children learn how to cope with the negatives in life. If a parent is always right, a child simply misses out on a huge part of learning. Confusing though it may seem, being wrong on occasions is the right way to parent.

As the parent of an IVF-conceived child, how do you ensure you are a 'good enough' parent? The two main strategies to employ are: firstly, to find good-quality parenting information and, secondly, to put yourself in your child's position when you consider parenting options, asking, 'What would I want a parent to do for me?'

Finding good sources of parenting information that you trust can be a tall order at times. There is no doubt you will be swamped with advice from all quarters from the time you announce the pregnancy. People love to tell you what they have learned or even what they think you should do in any given situation. Much of this information is conflicting, sometimes it is hurtful and often it is of little use.

Ideally, there would be an organisation in each country researching the parenting of IVF-conceived children to provide definitive answers about what techniques work for children and what doesn't. But many governments do have valuable information services for all parents (see Useful Contacts, page 201). Health-care professionals are also wonderful sources of information when families are struggling with anxiety or particularly difficult parenting issues. Family doctors, early childhood nurses, counselling professionals and developmental psychologists can all provide reassurance for parents. These professionals can also teach a healthy set of problem-solving skills that may help parents feel better supported.

Other parents who have successfully negotiated situations like yours are also an immensely valuable source of support and help. Just hearing someone say 'I felt just the same' can make your issues seem like small hills to climb and not the world's tallest mountain. Other parents who have older children conceived through IVF can be wise counsel to put your issues into perspective. You may be worried about your child's behaviour at two and hear that the parents of a ten-year-old found just the same, but the ten-year-old doesn't have tantrums any longer. Suddenly problems you feel are insurmountable fade away to become simply stages in a journey to successful parenting. See Useful Contacts, page 201, for information about finding IVF parent support groups.

The second part of being a good enough parent is being able to show empathy, to be able to ask yourself 'What would I want if I were a child?' Many difficulties can be readily sorted if you are able to put yourself into your child's shoes. Having empathy helps you to look for the reasons behind the child's behaviour, rather than simply labelling the child. Empathy also helps you make better choices for your child.

Empathy is something we learn as children from our own parents. Each time we are sensitively handled, fed when hungry, comforted when frightened and listened to when we have worries, we are learning that others have empathy for us. This teaches us to think of others as we grow. If we are not well cared for and listened to as children, we may continue into adulthood finding it hard to think of another as we become very self-focused. This trait makes good parenting more difficult.

Often self-focused people remember little of their childhood. I often ask parents struggling with difficult child behaviours to try to remember how they felt as children in stressful situations. For those parents who cannot find the memories, I always recommend a few sessions of individual counselling to help them get in touch with their childhood and perhaps process a few bad memories along the way. It may be painful at times, but it brings enormous rewards in terms of their ability to successfully and happily parent their own child.

For parents happy to remember childhood experiences, I ask them to describe their feelings when a parent told them off, when they made a mistake and when they were loved, comforted and understood. They invariably describe being traumatised by yelling or cold-hearted parents and finding it much easier to behave well when they were calmly dealt with. This is the blueprint to use for your own parenting. Set calm, firm limits on what is allowed, after a tantrum spend time with your child, who after all is still learning, gently explaining how the situation could be changed, praise your child's positive behaviours and ensure he feels unconditional love no matter his mood or behaviour.

Post-natal depression

One of the most common and testing issues young families face is that of post-natal depression (PND). Most people have heard of this term thanks to the awareness raised by national depression organisations and by celebrities such as Brooke Shields. Few people know exactly what PND means to new families and just how much distress it can cause.

In most cases, it is the mother who is diagnosed with PND, usually between three and twelve months after the birth. On occasions, a father may also be diagnosed with PND. What is crucial to understand about PND is that the whole family facing PND needs help. There should be no blame attached to any one family member nor should any member be singled out as 'the one with the problem.'

Studies have shown that as many as one in six mums may suffer PND; however the rate of PND amongst IVF mothers may well be higher. A 2005 study published in the journal *Fertility and Sterility* suggested that the incidence of PND may be as much as four times higher among IVF mums than non-IVF mums[1]. The occurrence in fathers is much harder to gauge as often the mother will seek help herself before her partner can be diagnosed. Furthermore, men are often more reluctant to seek professional help than women. I suspect the rate is higher for those using IVF — somewhere between 25 to 30 per cent of families — and research is beginning to support my view. The prevalence of PND among parents conceiving through IVF is a result of the intense anxiety the treatment process brings, added to the grief of infertility and the distancing that may occur in the couple's relationship. IVF families come to the early years of parenting already stressed and with too little in reserve to negotiate the hurdles of the early years with moods intact.

Families with PND often seem fine from the outside, but in reality are unable to function well. The mother (and father too) may show signs of exhaustion, intense anxiety and feeling everything is wrong. Those suffering from PND may also feel they are being chronically inadequate as a parent. There is often an instinctive 'survival mode' adopted when PND strikes. Parents do what has to be done, but there are no joyous moments, no spontaneous warmth, no great moments of interaction between parents, and no child-like play with all members of the family joining in. A parent's problem can affect the children's development and emotional well-being.

PND is fully treatable and requires sensitive and speedy help. Like most psychological illnesses, there is often much shame and guilt attached to having the disorder. Treatment is based around a family approach on a number of fronts.

An isolation 'cure'

Isolation is a problem most new parents face. You have left behind the days of being free (or perhaps having one child), and the activities that go with a childfree life. Both parents may leave work permanently or for a time, leaving a hole where once existed status, a sense of belonging and the existence of a group with shared goals. Many couples say they suddenly found good friends without children stayed away once the baby arrived, not wanting to get involved with nappies, feeds and early nights. More importantly, exhaustion may prevent either partner keeping in touch with friends and family in a way that is meaningful. And many parents who have struggled through IVF say they just feel 'different' and 'uncomfortable' with those who have no idea of their experiences and may even be frightened of them. The end result can be isolation and PND.

Reducing isolation must be a goal for all families who have been through IVF, especially when PND has been diagnosed. Isolation is the factor that constantly stands out in IVF research for its ability to harm the psyche. The more you can be comfortable with your route to birth, the better. Talking about how your baby was conceived, as a profoundly positive experience, may not be an easy discussion to have with others, yet being open about the process seems to protect against PND. Furthermore, your acceptance of the IVF route, and the openness with which you discuss it, has immense benefits for your children. Parents who are comfortable and honest about this will pass on this comfort to the children. You want a positive self-image for your children and they can certainly build self-esteem by seeing their conception as a positive experience.

You can come to an acceptance and openness about using IVF as loudly or as quietly as you wish. There are companies and organisations, primarily in the USA, that produce baby garments with IVF slogans or pictures (they are available online). This may not be everyone's idea of ending isolation but it certainly begins conversations. For a more subtle approach, parents can, from the beginning, refer to their baby by a nickname referencing the IVF process: for example, parents have called babies in the womb Number One, to reflect the best embryo chosen for implantation, or Cryo, for a successful frozen embryo. You can be as inventive as you like and humour helps too. The main idea of this is to make you both, and those around you, feel entirely comfortable with the technology that has brought you a family.

An essential part of ending isolation is getting to know other IVF families as social partners and information suppliers. Just as mothers' groups are intended to assist women help each other, so IVF parents need to set up their own support groups. There are several ways to create a group to meet your needs for meaningful support. You could contact your local newspaper and ask it to write about the need for a group of parents using IVF to meet and support each other. You can also contact your family doctor and ask for a notice to be put on the practice noticeboard. A third route is to advertise the group in the local baby clinic or parenting centre. Or you can join one of the IVF online forums and ask for local families to contact you (see Useful Contacts, page 201).

Coping with setbacks

My experience of working with parents who have conceived using IVF is that the stress and anxiety that the procedures create can often lead to parents feeling that 'everything will go wrong' no matter that they now have a healthy baby. Many couples have undergone many tests discovering fertility problems, a number of IVF cycles that did not work and have a slightly more pessimistic view of life as a result. Such experiences can create difficult feelings that ensure that every mild illness, every vaccination and every normal check a baby has produces intense anxiety for parents. Chronic anxiety forms the basis of one type of PND.

Parents can help themselves feel more positive over the early years by engaging a supportive family doctor. This is crucial for all anxious parents, however they have conceived. As new IVF parents, the best way to allay fears over your child's health is to have a supportive and encouraging doctor who provides the reassurance you need rather than belittling your concerns.

Ask your doctor for monthly visits at first to address any concerns you are having with your child and with parenting in general. Even if your questions seem odd to you, a good family doctor should sense you are anxious and be able to reassure you. It is also important to discuss any medical concerns, such as the possibility of any reaction your child may have to vaccinations and how to deal with this.

Achieving a team mentality

PND can be avoided, or treated if it does occur, by building a strong team spirit between you, as new parents. Just as the great sporting teams take team bonding very seriously, so must you as parents. A strong bond supports both of you in a healthy way, reducing the impact of the ups and downs encountered in parenting young children.

First and foremost, you are a couple and it is this bond, based on love and mutual respect, that builds a strong and lasting parenting team. Maintaining this bond requires regular time spent together without the added pressure of parenting chores.

In the early days, finding time to be alone as a couple can be a difficult task, particularly if you are the proud parents of multiples. A few simple ideas make the process a reality. Ask a friend or relative to come over during nap time and leave the baby monitor with him or her, then go out into your garden or balcony and have a quiet coffee and chat together — but ensure there is only positive talk, with no nagging allowed, and use the time to hold hands and enjoy each other's company. Have someone take the baby out in the pram, while you take twenty minutes out to enjoy each other over a snack in a café — people close to young parents are very happy to help in a way that has obvious benefits for the family as a whole.

As you become more comfortable leaving the baby with a responsible carer, take it in turns to plan dates. Most parents I counsel look aghast when I suggest this, as though dating were reserved solely for teenagers. A loving and respectful relationship requires constant effort to maintain the energy of the bond between you. Without this, the relationship withers and nagging problems surface, which take away the enjoyment of being together. Take time to be just a couple again, knowing your child will also benefit from the team spirit you generate.

Separation

A significant number of research studies have found that parents who have conceived their baby through IVF tend to have greater difficulty separating from a child than parents who have conceived naturally. This is because of the IVF parents' increased need to protect their child from danger, believing that only continual contact between parent and child will ensure survival. This anxiety means parents are unable to take a break, they may often quarrel with each other over who has the child's welfare most in mind, and they can become hyper-vigilant to danger. These three factors most certainly contribute to PND.

The best treatment for parental separation anxiety is to learn to face the fear just for a few moments at a time. This is a technique adapted from a process psychologists call systematic desensitisation.

First, I suggest to a parent, who is finding it hard to leave a baby with his or her partner, to begin separating very slowly. Allow your partner to hold the baby while you go into another room. Focus on taking deep breaths for five minutes then return. Gradually extend time away to ten minutes, then fifteen on consecutive days, until you can go into the garden or into the shower for thirty minutes. If, on a given day, you feel panic and cannot continue, simply accept this and continue your plan the next day.

Once you feel comfortable, take a five-minute walk away from home, deep breathing as you go. Increase this by five minutes once you feel confident about coping. Be assured that even if the baby cries, this will not hurt her at all, and in fact the realisation that she can be fine with other people is a normal developmental task to be accomplished. Once you are able, go shopping for half an hour, then repeat this whole process with your most trusted friend or family member instead of your partner. Once you have mastered this art, you can take a short break as a couple, leaving your baby safe in the knowledge that she is being well cared for.

The next big separation milestone for parents and children is day care or preschool. This can be handled in a similar way as the initial separation from your child: by taking time to familiarise yourself with the centre for a short period at first. Once you have mastered visiting the centre with your child for an hour, you can then gradually extend the periods that you leave him, asking that you be allowed to call the centre at regular intervals to check that he is settling. Some children do take time to get used to group environments without a parent present, particularly first children. The best method to help anxious children is to try short mornings twice a week. Provide lots of reassurance for your child, both when you leave him and when you return. In time, he will understand that you always come to collect him and his anxiety will ease.

There are suggested 'dos' and 'don'ts' to the timing of placing your child in care and, if followed, they will reassure parents they are not harming their children. Research has shown that day care can raise stress levels for children, in some circumstances making them vulnerable to behavioural problems.[2] Experts suggest that a baby is better cared for in the home by one or two people for the first year of life. I suggest a nanny share or family day care is used, if possible, for babies whose parents both work. It is also wise to have one parent with the child for the majority of the time, so perhaps working no more than twenty-five hours a week to start with is a good option for one parent, if you can afford it. An alternative could be if both parents could work on different days.

The internet has spawned massive growth in so-called 'mummy businesses', designed to provide a career that is manageable with childcare. Mothers the world over are amazingly creative, using career skills gained before having children, to launch new businesses. An AXA-sponsored survey in the UK in 2006 found that as many as 34 per cent of new and expectant mums seek to set up businesses from home. The benefits of home-based work include flexibility, being 'the boss' and avoiding the nightmare of asking for days off when a child is ill. As children get older, the parent can use day care for short periods to enable her to focus on the business while a toddler has time to socialise..

Between the ages of one and three, day care is helpful for two to three short days per week. It is wise to take time to reflect on your child's temperament before selecting a day-care centre. If your child is quiet and shy, find a small centre with warm, empathic staff. If your child is more of an extrovert, she may be happier in a setting where there are more children of her own age and opportunities for play with peers.

Parents who are anxious that they are giving insufficient attention to their children because of work can be reassured by following certain guidelines. The most important indicator that all is well with a child is that he is generally settled and behaves in a similar fashion through the week as he does at weekends. Children who are getting too little parental involvement will regularly use attention-seeking behaviours, such as tantrums, clinging, whining and engaging in behaviour that has been forbidden. They will be upset and possibly difficult on workday mornings and upset in the evenings when parents come home. These children may also sleep poorly.

For you as parents, there are also indicators that you are working too much. Are you desperate for your child to go to bed as soon as you get home? Have you lost your ability to be spontaneous with her? Do you find yourself nagging her more than you engage in positive interactions with her? If the answer to any of these questions is usually 'yes', consider trying to rearrange your working hours.

If you are a working father and feel you are missing out on bonding with your child, there are a few ways you can increase the connection between the two of you and feel less guilty. I suggest to couples that the father has a ritual morning with the child on Saturdays while the mother takes a break.

Dad can begin by staying at home with the baby while perhaps she goes out shopping. As the child grows, he can organise swimming or gym classes to attend with his child, with a stop for a drink or lunch and a little bonding on the way home. This bonding time will help him avoid depression and it will also lead to less friction between partners who have different ideas about how to care for their child.

Have fun

Pleasure is a necessary part of being healthy. The brain functions best when there are lighter moments to enjoy between intense bouts of obligation. Without pleasure, our moods become darker and we begin to look at life far too seriously. PND can easily be the result for parents of young children.

Parents who are very busy and anxious tend to put fun behind sleep, childcare duties, work, family duties, housekeeping and shopping. Fun is taken only when all other obligations have been attended to, which often means it does not happen. Over the first two or three years of parenting, the amount of seriously hard work increases as teething comes along, followed by illness, bouts of separation anxiety and toilet training. At the same time, the fun side of the equation may become very small and often non-existent. To be happy and healthy, fun time must at least equal serious time — preferably with an overspill.

Despite the numerous obligations of work, home, childcare duties and cooking, you can have fun with your child in tow without this becoming a chore. Soft play centres are great places to help your child become more sociable and to enable her to practise her motor skills too. As children get a little more independent, you can sit nearby and enjoy a coffee with other parents while keeping an eye on them.

Find nature every other weekend. Young children adore being in the open air and having some freedom. Go on a bush walk, find beautiful gardens to visit or take a picnic to a park and relax. The more you engage in relaxed outdoor activities with your children, the more they will enjoy them. Even if the preparation is hard before you get there, remind each other not to give up.

In summer, find a local pool, beach or river to enjoy a family day out in the water. It is hard not to shake off the cares of the world and indulge in a little fun when you're playing with water. Letting go of everyday stresses and strains helps parent-child bonding enormously, and it also reduces the level of stress hormones flooding the body. Avoid spending all your time instructing your child in how to swim – remember having fun makes learning new skills much quicker.

Visit animals regularly. Children love watching and petting animals and are often at their happiest with a day out at a zoo, aquarium or animal park. Stay only as long as it is enjoyable: different ages mean different concentration spans.

Take ten minutes each day to engage in spontaneous fun play with a child. With busy schedules, life can sometimes become a series of attempts to keep a child quiet while parents finish daily tasks. As stressed parents, make a promise to each other to take ten minutes, perhaps each afternoon, to play dress-up, trains, even a simple game of peek-a-boo with a one-year-old. This will increase your pleasure in life, as well as adding to your child's sense of well-being.

Parenting multiple children

Most parents of multiples speak of the first year in hushed tones, amazed they survived. They also feel very special and very much in awe of all they have achieved. 'I was very proud to tell people they were great babies and very easy to look after, even if there were two of them,' one mother said.

Parents also report multiples bring endless fascination. Watching babies grow together, interact and establish different identities is an amazing experience. 'It is so delightful to have two gorgeous babies at once,' a mother of twins said. 'Watching them play together and be together is fantastic. We have a boy and girl, so seeing gender differences is also interesting.'

As new parents of multiples, there are a number of pitfalls you need to be aware of in the early years. You can take steps to ensure you navigate the stress successfully, which is important since anxiety and post-natal depression are more common in parents giving birth to multiples through IVF. Obviously, having more than one baby at a time creates a great deal of work.[3, 4] Parents have less sleep and it is harder to take any form of time out, sometimes leading to chronic stress and sleep deprivation, two common precursors to PND. 'We are exhausted most of the time,' parents of twins said.

Sleeping habits

Sleep is usually uppermost on the minds of parents with multiples during the first year. The brain needs sleep to process traumatic events and to bring acceptance and resolution of fears. Inadequate sleep halts this function and parents can easily become 'stuck', focused on the anxiety something will go terribly wrong.

From three months onwards, the goals are to establish good sleeping habits, locate sources of reliable help, find other parents of multiples to share your experiences with and find time for positive and loving one-on-one parental interaction with your babies. From ten to twelve weeks, babies are much more able to self-settle. If your babies were born prematurely, self-settling will occur at their adjusted age — that is, the due date plus ten to twelve weeks. This is the time to try to put the babies in their cots awake but drowsy, to determine if they will be able to fall asleep by themselves.

Some multiples are able to self-settle in the same room; others are not. If your babies wake each other continuously, it may be wise to teach them to self-settle in separate rooms until they have mastered the art and can fall asleep together.

Parents of multiples can also suffer sleep issues when toddlers are moved into big beds. As they are now able to get out of bed unaided, they may be inclined to get together for a play date at bedtime. A firm but calm policy of taking them back to bed and saying nothing about 'bad behaviour' will often cure this problem. Star charts may also help, with each child getting a star for staying in bed at night. If one child is more tired than another, he can sleep while the other looks at picture books with a night light. The aim is to achieve a calm, predictable routine that offers little reward for toddlers who get up or wake a sibling.

Reliable help

The second important requirement for parents of multiples is sources of reliable help. Often, new parents are inundated with offers of assistance from fascinated friends and relatives in the first months after the birth.

But as the first few years go by, the offers are seldom followed up so diligently and parents whose children are into their third or fourth year often feel quite alone. This is a really crucial time to find dependable sources of help.

There are many potential sources of help, both paying and non-paying. As parents of more than one baby, you may wish to squeeze a little extra from the budget for the years until school begins and find some paid help. This provides you with reliability minus the guilt that you may feel asking for favours from friends. Part-time help from a college or a high school student can be a wonderful support, particularly at difficult times, including late afternoons, meal times and bath times. Such help can be found cheaply by putting notices in schools or colleges.

For free help in the form of multiple-sitting, you could join forces with other parents of multiples, or advertise for other parents of multiples through your family doctor. As multiple children pass babyhood, it is possible to have two sets of twins playing together for an hour once a week while one parent gets a break. Parents may also like to set up a multiples playgroup in their area so they can get together and take a little break while the children play.

Obviously, parents of 'higher order' multiples (three babies or more) face much greater problems in finding support because of the amount of work and costs generated. If you are the proud parents of higher order multiples, you may like to contact local colleges that run childcare courses, as students may require home placements for work experience. They will help alongside a parent for feeds and bath times and will usually come free. It is also a wonderful source of experience for the students.

Families and friends can provide help, and regularly do, but it is not an easy task for ageing parents to cope with two or more babies at a time. Grandparents can often be of more help caring for one child at a time, while a parent takes one or two children out with them. It is much easier to shop or run other errands with fewer children and one child will receive special one-on-one time with a beloved grandparent.

You will also find that spending time with other parents who are also discovering life with twins, triplets or more is a very important and wonderfully empowering act. Make contact with other parents through a multiple birth association (see page 202), and be prepared to go a little further from home in order to have a common understanding with other families. 'I have made some very good friends outside my area with multiple parents,' a mother of twins told me.

The individual children

The idea that multiples can be separated for a time and cared for by different people often comes as a surprise to parents of twins, triplets and more. Parents often see their multiples as one unit to be treated exactly the same. However, research with multiple children suggests some individuality is a sensible strategy to employ, as each child will have a different sense of independence and individual self-esteem. If you find outings with all your children can be exhausting, do not be afraid to take a child each on a Saturday morning if you are the parents of twins. The children love one-on-one time with a parent and it makes going out so much easier if you are responsible for only one child. The twins may miss each other but will quickly make up time when they are reunited. For the parents, one-on-one time encourages bonding with a child in a way that is difficult when siblings are together. This bond not only helps multiple children but also reduces stress for parents.

If you are the parents of triplets, leaving two children at home with one parent while taking it in turns to have one-on-one time with the third will foster strong bonds and reduce stress for the parent trying to run errands.

It can also be easier to play with two children at a time at home than to try to cater for the needs of three. Any guilt parents feel at separating the children can be answered by the fact that gaining individuality will foster a strong sense of self for all the children as they grow.

8

Where Do I Come From?

We saw the doctor who had done our treatment, and introduced
him to our boys.

Children begin to develop a sense of identity from the time they can
experience sounds, tastes and sensations in the womb. Creating an
identity continues during the first years of life, with the child needing
answers to the simple questions, 'Who am I? and 'Where do I come from?'

Such questions can pose difficulties for parents not accustomed to such
forthright demands from a very young child. Early questions about the
origins of life may be asked during the arrival of a younger sibling or a
friend's sibling. Questions continue, and become more complex during the
first years of school. Children are trying to make sense of the world and
how they fit into it. They also seek out similarities and differences between
their own families and those of their peers.

For parents who have conceived through IVF, there is added complexity
to the questions about identity. A child wanting to understand how she
came into the world may cause discomfort and even distress to parents
who have conceived using donor sperm, eggs or embryos, and the task of
helping a child create a healthy identity is a long, complex and somewhat
unknown path.

The identity questions require simple, sensible and truthful answers. However, children also need their parents to be comfortable and reassuring when discussing IVF and donor issues. You need to provide children with age-appropriate answers, as well as preparing yourselves to confront your own feelings about identity and IVF treatment.

'I'm normal, too'

Often, by the time couples have been through the intrusive IVF treatment, they feel anything but normal. The whole act of creating a baby is taken away from them and instead carried out by faceless scientists. It can be hard to avoid feeling like an alien from another planet. Parents often wonder how their child will feel about being conceived in this way.

It is very important that parents who have used IVF learn to accept the nature of conception. Parents also need to be able to talk about IVF with trusted friends and relatives, not to banish the subject because it is too confronting. As he grows, a child will need to be able to talk about where he came from, the miracle of his birth and issues over fertility that he may worry about. In order for parents to be fully supportive, they need to begin their discussions with each other over what they will say to their child long before he is ready to ask his first question.

Children use non-verbal communication, including facial expressions and body language, much more than they use words to determine whether they are being told the truth. So discussing conception with children not only needs the right words to be said in a positive way but also the use of positive body language. This is impossible if parents feel discomfort over the way their child was conceived.

The idea of becoming comfortable with IVF as a means of conception was discussed earlier (see pages 136–37), and the adoption of a special 'nickname' for a baby, or perhaps using baby clothes with IVF slogans, was suggested. Such ideas, with repetition, will help parents to feel relaxed and comfortable with IVF — even perhaps bored about the subject. Being able to talk to other families with IVF children will also reinforce that you are not unique in conceiving this way. Using IVF is no longer 'weird', and research shows the vast majority of people are now comfortable with the way this technology works, whether they have used it or not.

It is important for you to know that many different research studies show no significant cognitive or behavioural differences between IVF-conceived and naturally conceived school-aged children. A report published in 2004 stated that all available evidence showed the same psychosocial and academic outcomes for children, whether conceived naturally or by artificial reproductive techniques.[1] There may be a slightly elevated risk of illness and prematurity for IVF babies, but for those babies born without complications IVF parents can expect their children to have a very normal childhood. Furthermore, with the news in 2006 that the first test-tube baby Louise Brown had given birth to a son conceived naturally, IVF parents can expect that fertility will not be any greater issue for IVF children than it is for naturally conceived children. These very positive findings should help parents feel reassured when they come to talk about IVF with their children.

When to tell

Experts in the field of adoption have long implored parents not to wait to tell a child about his identity until he finds out from someone else. For a child, discovering this when parents are not there to help is devastating. I have worked with several adults who were adopted, but not told about it until a chance comment in the primary-school years led them to realise their origins. They reported being shocked and upset at first, feeling that their worlds were being turned upside-down. Psychological research reports that adopted children who discover their origins by accident instantly lose the sense of trust they had formerly developed with their adoptive parents.

With these experiences in mind, experts now recommend that, from an early stage, parents are honest with their children about their origins, whether a child has been adopted, or conceived through IVF using the parents' own embryo or with the involvement of a donor.

Opinion is divided over whether children should know their origins as soon as they are born or whether they should be told when they are a little older and can understand more complex concepts. There is certainly a case for telling children where they come from, in simple terms, very early in life. As children begin to develop their identity even before they are born, delaying the truth may lead to an older child being shocked at the disclosure and needing to significantly change the identity he has created. A much younger child will not yet have constructed much of an identity, and disclosure at a very early age may save the child some degree of pain.

'We are pregnant ...'

My personal belief about disclosure is that facing the issue even before birth is the best option. This method ensures there will not be a big occasion where stressful news is imparted in a highly charged atmosphere. Such a 'talk' can make the child feel frightened of what is coming and perhaps more traumatised than he needs to be.

As a couple conceiving through IVF, the advantages of talking to your baby about how he was conceived before he is even born are many. Before your baby has even learned how to be scared, he hears your voice, the intonation of your words and feels safe when you tell him many times of the miracle that created him (and you get used to talking about it). Unborn babies are amazing, and he will recognise the words you have repeated.

Your baby will come into the world accepting the wonderful way he was conceived before he even takes his first breath. IVF becomes part of his very core, a very acceptable part of who he is, and an issue that is never contentious or painful.

I couldn't say it before ...

Once your child has been born, the best plan is to tell her as soon as you both have a good opportunity, at a time when there are no other difficult issues on the horizon (see below). A child will find the news harder to deal with if she is already struggling. Avoid imparting the news around the time of starting preschool or school or near the birth of a sibling.

Before you decide on an opportunity to begin disclosure, you need to both come to an acceptance of the need to do so. If you remain unconvinced about the need to tell your child, try to imagine yourself as an eight- or nine-year-old child. You may suddenly learn about your origins by chance when a relative blurts out the truth. Suddenly you are told about an all-important event that deeply affects you and happened before your birth which no one had dared to mention before. By this stage of your life, you would have made assumptions about your origins, your family and how you fit into the world. A change in that perception after new information is provided can seriously destabilise a child for a time. I believe most children discovering a secret by accident would rather have known the story of their 'miracle' conception at an earlier age.

As parents, if you cannot agree about disclosure, or you both feel ashamed or embarrassed to talk about it, I suggest both attend a few sessions of counselling with an infertility counsellor, who is experienced in counselling parents after assisted conception. Even if you do agree about the need to tell your child, a few sessions of counselling can be beneficial to help you both come to an agreement of how best to approach the subject. Counselling also provides a useful opportunity for you to rehearse how you will explain IVF to your child.

Identity and IVF

In order to understand how to impart important conception information to young children, you need to understand how they build an identity and come to feel safe and competent in the world. Identity is a highly important issue: from a good sense of self, children can derive significant self-esteem throughout their lives and that will help them deal with any 'knocks' they suffer. A healthy sense of identity builds resilience.

The first people a baby forms relationships with are critical to both his short-term safety and long-term psychological well-being. Babies are primed with many different skills at birth that help them form close relations with others. For example, consider the way a day-old baby mimics a parent's speech and how quickly a two-month-old learns the art of taking turns during a conversation. Parents have an enormous ability to influence their child's trust and sense of identity in all their interactions. Parents also have significant influence on the way the child receives the news about his conception.

Modern psychology teaches us that babies and children move through different stages in their emotional growth. As parents ready to disclose important information, you need to understand the issues your child is struggling to master at any given stage and, consequently, the information he requires from you to keep him safe.

Before birth

I always talk to parents expecting the arrival of an IVF baby about the need to feel comfortable with the process they have used to conceive. IVF can be a taboo subject in social circles simply because people, who have not been through the treatment, do not know what to say. This encourages IVF parents to keep silent about their treatment, feeling a little embarrassed.

Such embarrassment is best worked on during the pregnancy because difficult feelings about the conception hinder the way parents tell their child, 'This is where you came from.' I always stress the benefits of being open and honest about IVF from the beginning so that the child always feels comfortable.

This does not mean IVF parents have to shout their method of conception from the rooftops! I simply suggest that parents awaiting their child talk about IVF with a few close friends and family members who can be trusted to keep confidences. This helps parents to feel more comfortable and accepting of their child's conception.

As a newborn

Once your baby arrives, continue to talk honestly with your chosen confidantes. Discuss the topic of IVF on occasions, how it has changed your life and how it has also impacted upon it in a difficult way. This continues to help you feel comfortable with IVF so that, in turn, your baby can feel comfortable as she grows.

I also suggest to new IVF parents who are having an emotional time after the birth to talk over their feelings with a professional counsellor. Fears over the use of IVF and about how to tell your child about conception when the time comes are best dealt with in the early days of parenting as this also prevents stress affecting your baby.

As a toddler

The toddler years bring a wonderful, though at times confronting, sense of autonomy and the ability to say 'no' frequently. Throughout this stage, children are learning that they are independent little people with likes and dislikes, and with the ability to make others listen to them. Toddlers need lots of calm reassurance that even though they can assert their wills, and even lose control in a tantrum, ultimately they are always loved by their parents.

This is the stage where compiling a photo diary of the pregnancy, birth and early months is helpful. Toddlers love to see pictures of their parents and of themselves as babies, ultrasound pictures of them as a baby growing in the womb and photos of their parents during pregnancy. Using the pictures, you can explain that Mummy and Daddy went to a special place where doctors help lots of people make babies. Describe how you had to go to the clinic a lot of times and the doctors helped you make a baby, and when she was tucked up in Mummy's tummy to grow you were so excited. Try to tell the story in much the same way every time you discuss the subject. The photo diary can be given to your child to keep safely when she is older.

As a young child

The preschool years are full of accomplishment, as the child begins to master skills that help her socialise, play and learn. Positive praise for all that she does well at this stage is highly important, added to firm limits that are calmly explained and consistently enforced. Criticism from parents at this stage can easily make a child feel guilty, just as confusing explanations of a child's origins, impatiently told, can induce guilt. As IVF parents, ensure you take the time to consider your child's questions appropriately and if you cannot answer right away, make a specific time with your child to talk later in the day.

This is the time when storytelling becomes highly important for imparting information to a child, And it is an ideal way of giving her a sense of where she came from. For parents at ease with their IVF treatment, I recommend developing your own stories of how your child came to be, adding to these stories a little more information each time. Children are very easy to read in terms of how much information they need at a particular point. Tell your child the very basics and leave her for a few days. If she needs any more information, she will raise the subject, asking further questions. If no questions are asked, you can be assured that for the time being at least she is satisfied with the information you have given her.

At this stage, when preschoolers see friends with new baby siblings or a friend's mother who is pregnant, they are curious about where babies come from. It is wise to talk to them about how families are all similar in some ways but are different in others. One family may have a single mother, another may have much older children or be a blended family. Children of this age can appreciate that differences do exist — and that these differences do not change how nice or how acceptable people are. This is a good point to discuss as a family: your child has been conceived with a little extra help, other children in her preschool class may have been conceived in a different way, but all children are equal and just as loveable no matter how they came into being.

If you find it hard to discuss the way your child was conceived now that she is more knowing, you may find it easier to read her a story. There are a few good storybooks available that you can use to ease the process. The best of these is one designed especially for children conceived through IVF: *The Story of an IVF Baby* in the 'X, Y and Me' series by Janice Grimes. Grimes is a nurse at an American IVF clinic and her wonderfully observant yet simple take on the concept will delight parents and children alike.

As an older child

The primary school years mark the stage when the child is learning to feel capable socially, academically and physically. Children of this age very much want to fit in with their peers. They are becoming much more aware of being an individual, yet at the same time realise they are part of a community. The goal for parents is to provide a rock-solid base from which the child can venture into the world a little at a time, returning to share both successes and hurts with his caring parents.

In terms of his origins, a child of this age conceived through IVF needs more information. It is during these years that school discussions covering the topic 'Where do I come from?' prompt questions from children such as 'Am I different?' and 'Will people know what happened before I was born?' Reassurance is needed in large quantities. For example: you may tell your child, 'You are just the same as all your friends. You began as a sperm and an egg that joined together like everyone else, you are made up of cells just the same as anyone else, you have a brain just the same, you look the same and you have a normal birthday just like everyone else. The only difference between all your friends is that some parents may have had a baby easily but others need some help. You won't be able to tell which parents needed help and which did not.'

Some children may tell close friends, perhaps proudly, that they are special and needed special doctors to come into the world. Other children may say nothing. As long as the subject is raised at appropriate times within the family and there is no code of silence about IVF, children will use the information about their conception in the way that suits them best.

As a teenager

The high school years mark a new phase of intense identity searching. Most teenagers desperately want to fit into their peer group and any issue that makes them feel different can be hard to accept. These years are often tumultuous in many ways, in any case, and it is unlikely that teenagers previously told they were conceived with IVF will have any greater conflicts to deal with than their naturally conceived peers. Indeed, early studies reporting IVF teens' experiences reveal very little differences between the issues that concern them and those with which all teens wrestle.

By this stage, teenagers need to know more about their origins and will use the information not just to describe 'Who I am now' but also to ask 'How will this affect me?' As the parents of an IVF-conceived teenager, you are likely to face more personal questions about the treatment process, especially as IVF is often talked about in the media. You may not wish to disclose very personal features of IVF treatment, such as 'Dad and I tried for five years ...', even though teens are often very curious about their parents' personal experiences. Instead, you can talk in general terms along the lines of 'Many people find ...' This way you protect your own privacy while giving your teen the information she needs.

Teenagers are remarkably good at searching for answers and do not always rely on their parents for information. Peers, books and the internet all provide information required to more easily define the IVF process and what this means to a teenager. As you parent your IVF teenager, make it clear that it is natural for her to ask you questions and be prepared to do a little searching on the internet yourself if you are not totally sure of all your answers. It is not always being right that is crucial, but always being available for a teenager brings the most benefit.

As they become interested in members of the opposite sex, some teenagers may begin to ask questions about how IVF affects their appeal to partners. It is important to reassure them that they may never know whether or not a particular friend at school was conceived naturally unless the information is supplied by the teenager or parent concerned. In the same way, no one will know that IVF was part of your teen's conception unless she wants to impart the information.

Teenagers may also wonder if they will suffer fertility issues too, since some fertility problems are of genetic origin and can be passed from one generation to the next. In the future, it will be increasingly possible to test for these anomalies, perhaps even during the IVF process, to ensure infertility is not passed on from parent to child. In the meantime, the evidence from the first IVF successes is that the use of IVF itself does not lead to infertility problems for adults conceived through the process. This can be encouraging news for teenagers. However, a genetic fertility problem that required the use of IVF for a couple to conceive may be passed on to a child, who may also require IVF to conceive. If teens are worried about this, it is worth investigating any simple tests that can be done to reassure them.

At the teen stage, it is also important for both girls and boys to understand that fertility is limited by age as well as by physical problems, such as blocked tubes or low motility sperm. Teenagers need to understand that media portrayals of powerful working couples in their thirties 'having it all' with the perfect family are not always reality. As a species, we have spent a great deal of time and money convincing ourselves that we can achieve anything with effort and scientific input. Teenagers need to know that there are still many issues we do not control and that they cannot forget age when considering when to start a family.

Teenage girls, particularly, face a difficult time as they look into the future. Although women make up ever-larger numbers in the workforce, they are still the main caregivers of their children. Part-time work of many different varieties is still the norm for most mothers while their children are small; even later, teenagers can often require more care than two full-time working parents can provide. Women still feel very much that they have to make the choice between career and family at certain stages of their children's development.

It is important that both parents are able to talk to their children about issues involved in having a family. Such issues may include the choices parents made, their feelings about these choices and the different options they may have considered but not used. It is also important not to force parental opinions on to children; instead, IVF parents need to offer children their experiences, together with good information, and leave them to make up their own minds.

You're like me

By the time IVF babies conceived this year reach school age, it is likely that there will be one IVF-conceived child in every class in every school. Increasingly, IVF-conceived children will have similarly conceived peers to reinforce the fact that they are not unique.

Until this time, children can be helped to understand they are not 'freaks' by getting together with other IVF-conceived children. Establishing a network of IVF families who support each other will be important, not just for the early years but also for the years of cognitive development when older children and teens are learning all about the complexities of the world. Parents can tell a child they are not unique, but seeing this is better than being told, and meeting with another IVF child or teen will be valuable in proving this point. This is another area where support groups of IVF parents will really assist children to grow up accepting the truth that they are just like lots of other kids.

Issues over identity do not cease to become important when a child passes his eighteenth birthday and legally becomes an adult. The twenties and thirties mark a new phase in identity-searching as people find partners and have families. The younger years and the ability of parents to help their children grow to be comfortable and secure in their origins will affect the adult at this time.

There is scant information about IVF children who are now adults and how they react: few IVF births occurred before the mid 1980s. Although Louise Brown has just become a mother herself, little is known about her feelings on the subject, apart from expressions of delight from both Louise and her partner now that they have a son.

In time, studies of IVF children will follow these groups into adulthood and record their difficulties and triumphs. We will have a much better understanding of the feelings IVF-conceived adults have on becoming parents themselves, together with highly useful information regarding the methods of conception that were used. We can then base professional advice to prospective IVF parents on these facts.

For now, we must rely on anecdotal evidence and a determination to ensure these adults have access to professional services should they require them. For this reason, I think it is psychologically prudent to offer couples pre-parenting counselling if one or both partners were conceived through IVF. Such help would offer the chance for both prospective parents to consider their feelings about IVF and about the many other facets of the parenting role they are about to assume. It will ensure that any lingering doubts or fears they may have experienced earlier in their lives are brought out in the open, discussed and shared, thereby allowing them to focus their thoughts on their unborn baby without distraction.

The donor question

Parents of children conceived through IVF from donated eggs, sperm or embryos face the identity issues that all IVF parents face. But the presence of a donor in the parenting equation poses additional concerns that must be addressed.

About one-third of donor conceptions are because of female infertility, one-third through male infertility and one-third are for unexplained reasons. The level of difficulty families face in each situation is not equal, however, since much research indicates male infertility is a harder issue to confront than any other.

There is a much greater likelihood that a couple who used a sperm donor will maintain a silence about the method of conception than if a donor egg had been used. A number of reasons have been suggested for this. Men tend to define their whole beings, and therefore derive great self-esteem, from their virility. Fertility is associated very closely with virility. Many men still describe themselves as 'less of a partner' in a relationship if they are diagnosed as infertile. They feel somehow weakened and less able to provide for a mate. Thus, there is a strong reason for both partners to maintain a dignified silence about infertility.

Men also have less of a role in pregnancy and cannot 'make up' for their lack of input into conception, as women do. Many women using donor eggs, though they may well have some uneasy feelings, rarely feel the disconnection from the pregnancy that men feel. And it may be that male partners need much more time to bond with a baby conceived through a donor than the female partner needs. Although women do have misgivings over the use of a donor egg, such reactions are usually less intense than men's.

It is common for both partners to wonder what the baby will look like with the involvement of a donor. Parents may ask themselves, 'Will people notice the baby's facial features and comment that they are different to ours?' They may worry that the child's hair colour, mannerisms and academic capabilities will be noticeably different from theirs. Parents may well be concerned about undesirable genetic traits which may not be identified in the selection process. They may worry about genetic weaknesses, such as medical complaints that are not yet screened for. Such misgivings are often overcome in pregnancy by partners being able to talk to each other and by both having access to counselling services. The birth is usually a highly reassuring time for parents of a donor-conceived baby and, most often, the niggling worries about differences that parents may feel during a pregnancy disappear as they fall in love with the baby they are caring for.

A telling time

Research has shown that, at the time of questioning, up to 25 per cent of parents were undecided about whether they would tell their child about the donor. More and more evidence is demonstrating the damage uncertainty and even secrecy over the use of a donor can do within families. In order to construct a stable identity for life, at an early age children need to have a very basic understanding of their origins. Parents, therefore, need an understanding of what they can do to help their child.

Health ethicist Professor Derek Morgan has described a condition known as 'genetic anger', the frustrations donor-assisted, IVF-conceived teens feel at the lack of knowledge they have of their biological parents' identities.[2] This anger can stem from not being told of the donor at an early age, when they are establishing their own identity, and from the lack of information on their genetic characteristics and origins, which are available to other teenagers.

IVF parents can address the first part of this so-called genetic anger: the lack of knowledge of donor involvement in conception. Just as we now urge adoptive parents to talk to their children from the very beginning about where they came from, so donor children need the same information. Children need this information so that they are able to construct the identity they have within their family and in the world. Although complex concepts take time to master, the truth should always be used, albeit in a very simple form, from the earliest opportunity.

Many parents who used donor insemination in the early days before IVF was developed were advised by experts to keep silent about the method of conception. It was felt better for all concerned if secrecy were maintained. We know now that such secrecy destroys trust and family stability, and can have serious consequences for the psychological well-being of a donor child for her entire life.

Donor children face a number of issues if the identity of their donor is not made available to them. The first issue donor teens often fear is that, without knowing the identity of a biological parent, they may become romantically involved with a half-sibling. This fear does not exist without foundation: in the earliest days of donor programs when secrecy was the norm, it is possible that a number of infertile couples living in the same city would have received sperm from the same unknown donor and that two of these resulting children could become romantically linked.

The second issue that results from donor secrecy is that children, and teens particularly, feel inconsistencies in the parent-child relationship that can give them a sense of being unsafe. Parents may leave gaps in their explanations to 'where did I come from' questions to avoid telling a child about the donor part of the process. Children quickly sense when something is missing and tend to invent far worse explanations for the discrepancy than the actual truth.

Parent-child mistrust may lead to a worsening of the parent-child relationship. Professor Ken Daniels, of the School of Social Work and Human Services at the University of Canterbury in New Zealand, undertook research to investigate such bonds. This showed that 'those mothers who had decided to keep the use of DI [donor identity] a secret were experiencing more difficulties with their children than those who had told or who were intending to tell.'[3, 4] Daniels proposes that secrecy over the use of a donor suggests parents are ashamed of what they have done. 'Feeling ashamed is not a good basis for a healthy family,' he concludes.

The third issue stemming from donor secrecy, and discussed by Daniels, is the tremendous lack of trust generated when children do find out they were conceived using a donor. A child loses trust in the parents who maintained the secrecy and he often fears there are additional 'big secrets' he is not being told. There can be a great deal of pain on both sides, with intense hostility felt by the child.

Many parents conceiving through the use of a donor fear the child will search for a 'real' parent and fail to bond with the parents who are raising them. Such a view is very natural; however, evidence strongly suggests that donor-conceived children who know their origins early on bond very happily with their parents. Research shows that the children trust the parents' explanations of who they are and that they do not turn away from these parents when they are old enough to search for information about the donor who helped create them. Their love for the parents who have raised them is not related to their need to discover the identity of the donor to whom they are biologically related. It appears to be the case that the more parents help their children find out about their origins, the stronger the bond that grows between them.

Ending the silence

Donor use is a somewhat difficult subject to broach for many parents, who often do not know how to begin. Children's storybooks on the subject are the most sensible method of introducing these issues to your child. As for all IVF-conceived children, you can begin reading stories when your unborn baby reaches about thirty weeks' gestation. The 'X, Y and Me' website is an excellent place for information about complex IVF-related issues, and you can obtain children's stories based on donor eggs, donor sperm and donor embryos. A British-based charity, The Donor Conception Network, have produced a series of booklets designed to help parents and children discuss donor issues. Called *Telling and Talking*, the booklets are written for four different age groups: up to seven years, eight to eleven years, twelve to sixteen years and over seventeen. The network has also produced a DVD of parents and children talking about donor issues, which can be of use to bewildered parents. Also, check to see if you can borrow children's storybooks about donor involvement from a donor conception support group. See Useful Contacts, page 201.

Once your donor-conceived baby is born, every so often read the stories about how she was created so that it becomes a familiar and very normal component of life. Each time you read the story, your child will understand a little bit more of the complexity of donor-assisted conception. There is no need to go into more detail than the book does, unless your child asks for more information, in which case keep it simple and wait to see if she needs to return with further questions. Processing of the information given takes time, and it is so important that your child sets her own pace of understanding. Rushing her can create unwanted and unnecessary anxiety.

The second component of donor child anger, which parents need to help older children to accept, is the lack of information available to those born through donor programs fifteen or twenty years ago. Information availability is dependent upon government legislation, since donors rarely submit identity information through choice. The legislation concerning donor identity, and consequently the amount of information available, varies from one country to the next.

For many teens and adults conceived using donor eggs, sperm or embryos, there is little available information regarding donor characteristics or medical history. In the early days of donor programs, many clinics filed the barest of details and some even destroyed the information after a few years. The anonymity is one of the reasons so many men donated sperm, feeling that after the donation the matter was finished. This lack of identity now leaves many donor-conceived individuals with huge question marks over who they are, where they came from and their genetic history. It is as though this question mark becomes a sore that aggravates and cannot be ignored, compelling a donor child to work towards discovering the truth. Many donor teens explain that they do not wish to turn their backs on the parents who raised them, nor do they necessarily want a long-term relationship with a donor. They simply need to know the biological part of their history in order to be able to accept themselves and to live a normal life. Often when these donor-conceived children grow up and have children of their own, these issues of identity once again become very important.

Identity is extremely important for donor children but has a significant negative effect on the number of available donors. Sperm donation, particularly, was commonplace years ago and many young men offered to donate sperm thinking this act was no more complicated than giving blood. Many then forgot about the donation completely, only realising recently, with increased media interest in donor issues, that there were potentially life-long issues arising from their selfless act. The effect has been to dramatically lower the number of willing donors. Donor centres have been forced to scale back the number of couples they are able to help and some have closed their doors completely.

Although we will never know for certain, donor identity laws may also reduce the number of donor eggs and embryos now available to infertile couples. Couples with frozen 'spare' embryos do not have the option to donate anonymously, but if they did have that right it is possible they may use this option. Protecting the rights of children, though, must come first and knowing donor identity is of the greatest importance in ensuring donor children become happy well-balanced adults.

Who am I now?

There is some published research available to help parents with children of varying ages who do not yet know about their donor origins. These parents want to know how best to help their children and what to expect if the children are told of the donor who helped in their conception. Initial research findings suggest the current recommendation that children should be told about their origins from an early age has not been followed.[5, 6] Around 30 per cent of parents interviewed after egg, sperm or embryo donation say they will never disclose the fact to their child. There appeared to be no greater numbers of fathers not wishing to tell than mothers.

But, according to the 30 per cent of parents who do tell their children at a young age, typically it was a very factual process rather than an emotional one. Children asked practical questions, allowing parents to gradually increase the amount of information supplied without fear. Perhaps a system of 'donor-parent buddies' — based around parents who have already told their donor children about their origins — can help brand-new donor-assisted families to explore the issues around telling and the benefits the practice can bring. New parents could ask questions and gain support, noting how 'normal' donor families are when the donor information has been disclosed.

One aspect of telling older children about donor issues is the fear of stigma. Parents are concerned their child may feel different and will be singled out for unwanted attention because of this difference. In reality, children who have good self-esteem will integrate well with other children, no matter what their origins. Healthy self-esteem will come from parents praising the child's unique gifts and supporting her to learn right from wrong without serious anger or fear. A healthy self-image will also result from parents ensuring a child feels they are right behind her, supporting her, without intruding into every aspect of her life. Donor children will also gain self-esteem from meeting other donor children and understanding there is no way to distinguish whether he was conceived using a donor or not. Parents can tell their child that she was wanted very much, they went through a long process to have her and she is loved unconditionally.

The current legal situation

Two thousand babies are born each year in the UK involving donor eggs, sperm or embryos. The legislation regarding donation has been changed recently with new laws coming into effect in 2005 that ensured any child born through the use of donation would be able to access information about the donor.

The UK's Human Fertilisation and Embryology Authority maintains a donor register to allow children to discover information about their donor parents once they reach the age of eighteen. Details that are maintained on the register include their name, date and place of birth and an address at the time of donation. Children born before 2005 will only be able to access donor information if it was supplied voluntarily at the time.

Information about successful pregnancies can also now be made available to donors. If you have donated eggs, sperm or embryos, you are now entitled to discover the number of children born, their sex and dates of birth. This is often welcome information for people who have made the very complex decision to donate and can now know just how much their donation has meant.

The legislation enacted in 2005 also sought to set a limit on the number of times a donor's eggs, sperm or embryos could be used. Such limits try to ensure that the likelihood of two related children unknowingly meet and fall in love. The law now provides for 10 families being able to use the same donor.

Full details of the current legislation are available from the Human Fertilisation and Embryology Authority whose address is in the 'Useful Contacts' section at the back of the book. Information and support is also available through an organisation set up to support donors and families, the Donor Conception Network. The contact for this organisation can also be found in the 'Useful Contacts' section.

9

A Controversial Future

I'm mum to two sets of twins and one little embryo still in storage.

That hot July day when the Browns welcomed baby Louise into the world marked a new beginning for many couples who experience infertility. Over the last three decades, the ground-breaking technology that enabled this milestone of the first 'test-tube' baby has had a most profound effect on the lives of millions of parents and children from all over the world.

Statistics reveal that there has been enormous growth in the number of IVF treatments performed in the last ten years. More importantly, there has been a doubling of the success rate of IVF in the last twenty years. It is undoubtedly true that the success achieved through IVF will break many more records in years to come.

However, the road ahead is not smooth. Success aside, IVF technology has also had its critics. In recent years, the technique has been at the centre of ethical dilemmas for doctors, scientists, lawyers and governments. The debates on what is in the best interests of each couple, each child and our species as a whole are continuing.

Is IVF safe?

Reports emerging from some fertility experts, including the British expert Robert Winston, warn that the technology has developed too quickly for rigorous studies to be carried out on the health outcomes for IVF parents and children. Although most countries hold databases that detail all the treatments carried out and success rates achieved, researchers have often not been granted access to these data in order to carry out follow-up studies of birth outcomes and the difficulties experienced by families as children grow. This balance is beginning to be addressed, but there are still few reliable studies that measure the safety of the treatment in all its forms, for both parents and children.

The strongest evidence to support the need to make IVF safer is emerging from data about the well-being of mothers given high doses of stimulating drugs. Studies appear to show that a number of problems occur during this phase of treatment, requiring medical care and, in some instances, hospitalisation: they include hyper-stimulation of the ovaries and ectopic pregnancy. The push towards 'soft IVF' techniques — that is, the use of far lower levels of ovary-stimulating drugs — will hopefully reduce the incidence of female medical abnormality. Soft IVF may also hold the key to increasing success rates for IVF treatment still further as there is some evidence to suggest that stimulation of the ovaries may well harm some of the eggs that are later harvested, leading to lower implantation rates.

A frozen legacy

The most controversial issue surrounding IVF is the existence of six million frozen embryos waiting in storage for decisions to be made about their futures.

Freezing 'spare' embryos has become a valuable and normal part of the IVF process. For couples going through ovarian stimulation prior to IVF, the ability to harvest many eggs and 'save' successful embryos for a later date provides enormous psychological benefits. There are also physical and financial benefits from freezing spare embryos, since this means women do not have to undergo further costly ovarian stimulation prior to fertilisation and implantation. Couples can use a frozen embryo if the first cycle fails, or they can use their saved embryos to achieve further pregnancies. Studies show embryos preserved up to thirteen years can still result in healthy pregnancies,[1] so most couples will have ample time to decide when to implant their 'spare embryos'.

But what happens to the embryos when couples decide their families are complete or that their repeated IVF attempts have taken too great a toll on their lives? At the present time, there are three ways that frozen embryos can be released from long-term preservation at the end of storage. Firstly, couples can elect to donate thawed embryos for research. Secondly, parents can donate embryos to other couples who cannot use their own. Finally, embryos can be discarded. Studies show that donation is not the most popular option, with most couples electing to discard embryos or donate them for medical research in the hope of helping to further enhance the IVF process.[2]

Governments in countries where IVF is used extensively are now beginning to legislate for maximum embryo storage periods, realising that the issue will be increasingly emotive as more and more embryos end up frozen and unused. In the UK, embryos can be maintained in storage for five years before disposal. Couples can apply at the end of the five years for an extension in certain circumstances. In the US, individual states implement legislation for maximum embryo storage times and this legislation varies considerably.

The difficulty of the decision facing couples who have frozen embryos is only now beginning to be documented and discussed as new legislation is forcing an end to storage. We are still a long way from properly supporting couples and providing them with psychologically prudent and well-researched advice. For the foreseeable future, the issues to be considered and openly discussed remain numerous and complex.

It is hard for parents to get unbiased guidance about what decision to make. Those who have not been through IVF may find it difficult to understand the feelings of parents about the fate of their embyros. Parents have often told me that relatives simply advised them to dispose of the embryos, saying, 'They are not alive yet, so don't feel bad.' Despite the good intentions of these advisors, they often cause a great deal of pain. I have seen couples' distress on learning that their embryos did not divide properly after fertilisation through IVF and that these embryos had to be discarded before implantation was even attempted. Frozen embryos, which are no longer useful, elicit similar feelings of ownership and loss. No matter how much science is involved in IVF, there is a great deal of unavoidable grief over a potential life that was not achieved. Such feelings must be noted, processed and, with expert professional help, allowed to fade naturally over time. Suppression of these very understandable emotions serves only to cloud a family's pleasure in having the children who were very much wanted.

Once parents agree to discard embryos or to donate them to other couples, there is no way back. They cannot change their minds a few years later and decide they are not comfortable about donating spare embryos that are now children being raised by other people.

In seeking advice about frozen embryos, parents may turn to the IVF clinic they used. Most clinics are the point of contact when the legal time limit for storage is reached. However, these clinics also often have couples on waiting lists for embryo donation. The professionals at these clinics, who are dealing with prospective parents, cannot give unbiased advice to couples making decisions about their frozen embryos.

Counselling professionals may be experienced in assisting people to talk through the moral dilemmas and in finding the best way through for the individuals concerned. However, few of these professionals are experienced in talking with families about such complex life-long decisions. Due to the newness of the dilemma, there is little professional research available for guidance.

Support groups are also sources of information in making complex decisions. However, individuals within these groups may have been donor parents or donor children themselves and have very strong views on the pros and cons of donation or destruction. Parents may feel they want to talk to someone who is completely unaffected by the problem.

As the number of frozen embryos grows and more laws are passed to regulate the time they can be stored, more and more parents will face the dilemma of what to do with their frozen embryos. Researchers need to compile a database of available research and put in place a network of trained counsellors working in the public health domain who can assist parents to make these decisions. Parents would then be able to trust that such counsellors will allow them to consider all options properly and to help them select the best option.

It is not realistic to expect parents to make such a decision without experiencing grief, guilt and other painful emotions. These emotions need to be aired, supported and worked through in the time each person needs to achieve comfort with the decision.

If parents opt to discard frozen embryos, there will be some sense of loss that these hard-fought potential lives never came to be. Parents may feel a sense of fear that letting these embryos go puts paid to the chances of another pregnancy, even if they believe their family is truly complete. This sense of loss is similar to the sense of loss felt by some parents after a vasectomy or tubal ligation; they do not want more children but losing the ability to have them can be a painful experience too.

Couples may also experience guilt that they have embryos to spare while other couples cannot conceive. This may be especially pronounced if they have friends or relatives who are experiencing infertility. Parents need to anticipate these difficult feelings but also realise that discussing them openly over a period of time will bring about some acceptance if they decide discarding embryos is the right decision.

The choice to donate embryos for research is again one that can bring complex emotions to the surface. Parents may feel they are helping other couples through research that improves the IVF technique and leads to greater success rates in the future. Religious beliefs also play a part in this decision: for some, the sanctity of life cannot be questioned and therefore experimenting with life is not an option. Parents considering donation for research must accept the embryos are not 'life' as they define a living being, but simply clusters of cells too premature to experience any facet of life. This option may also bring about a sense of loss because the ability to try another IVF cycle has been removed.

The decision to donate spare embryos to other couples brings difficult questions about relationships, both biological and emotional. Parents wonder how their children will cope with the idea that genetically related brothers and sisters exist but live with other families. More complex still is the issue of a donor child's right to have full information about the identity of donors. Many parents express the fear that donating embryos will result in children who they may never know about. But legislation in the next few years will enshrine a child's right to know his donor's identity, providing an opportunity to establish contact. Parents may struggle to cope with the vision of their eighteen-year-old donor child making contact, requesting a meeting and perhaps even wanting to consider himself 'part of the family'. It is hard to imagine how any member of the family would feel if this possibility became a reality: it is likely that children will find the situation every bit as emotionally confusing as their parents.

To donate embryos to other couples requires an acceptance that, once they are donated, the donors have no control of the embryos, they have no right to discover what became of them and no right to dictate whether or not their own identities are revealed. It is up to the donor child, and potentially the donor parents, to make contact if and when this is desired. Some couples are able to give up that control happily, in order to share their own joy of becoming a family with others.

In this instance, I believe, these parents are able to come to terms with their decision and this acceptance will be communicated to their children, resulting in a family capable of coping with a donor child who wants to meet them. These couples go on to be very happy, psychologically well-adjusted donors. But some couples simply cannot achieve this.

Other facets of human life complicate the options for frozen embryos that have been stored beyond the maximum time. There are instances when partners cannot agree on the fate of their frozen embryos: one parent may want to donate an embryo to another couple but the other partner cannot accept this. Such disagreements are particularly difficult if couples have divorced: such cases have been taken to court in America. Again, as time goes on and more embryos are frozen, governments may well step in, legislating that at the time their embryos are frozen all couples sign agreements determining what will happen to unused embryos in the future.

To have or have not?

Frozen embryos are only the first of many complex issues that IVF raises. IVF has been a substantial part of the reason why women are giving birth later in life. The UK's Office for National Statistics last year reported a 7 per cent increase in the fertility rate for British women aged 35 to 39, part of which is due to assisted conception. The US in 2006 also saw a rising fertility rate across all ages. With IVF births continuing to form a larger and larger proportion of all births in these countries, the fertility rates of older women especially may well continue to climb.

The fact that humans now live longer than ever before suggests that having babies later does not necessarily change the basic structure of the lives of parents or their children. We become adults, mate, have children, raise these offspring and send them out into the world as responsible adults, whether we have children at age twenty or at age forty-five. However, there are subtle differences with childrearing later in life that can create issues for families. Older parents have to face greater pressures, such as looking after elderly or unwell parents, who cannot assist with childcare. Among families I work with, the lack of grandparent care can lead to greater rates of post-natal depression and in more children attending day care from an early age. The impact of early day care is still not truly known.

For parents in their forties, pregnancy and new parenting is generally more exhausting than it is for younger parents. Mothers may find that it takes a substantially longer time to recover from the birth, to regain energy and to attain a comfortable body shape than it does for younger women. There are usually more work pressures, which can bring enormous consequences for those who wish to reduce hours or to take time away to care for a child. This can be exacerbated by the fact that 'forty-somethings' generally enjoy a higher standard of living than younger parents and find it harder to compromise on lifestyle when a baby comes along.

Although these issues are frustrating for some, many couples very happily parent in their forties. I do not believe that having a baby at forty-two will change much about the lives of parents or babies, providing that parents take care of their health as much as possible and recognise the need to find support from alternative sources if their own parents are unavailable.

The age issue, however, is more contentious when much older women have children. The trend in certain countries to offer IVF to ever-older women may well lead to very disturbing outcomes for both parent and child. The ramifications of this defiance of the natural childbearing age are yet to be revealed. At the time of writing, the oldest IVF mother, who gave birth to twins in Spain in January 2007, was sixty-six years old. Soon after the birth, she revealed that she had lied to IVF specialists in America, stating she was fifty-five, the maximum age at which clinics would provide treatment. It seems some clinics do set maximum age guidelines but may not be checking patient information thoroughly.

How will these twins fare when they are ten, fifteen or twenty-one years of age? If she is still alive, how will their mother cope with raising teenagers at the age of seventy-nine? Will she ever see her children reach adulthood? There is no research available on the effects of pregnancy for women in their fifties and sixties, and no data regarding the effects of stimulating drugs, labour and the child's early years on much older women. We have no information as to how the children cope with their parents: for example, whether these children will face psychological issues not experienced by their peers. These are questions that need urgent answers, so governments can set legal age limits for IVF clinics to follow.

A recent announcement of a 58 year old giving birth through IVF prompted the UK's Human Fertilisation and Embryology Authority to state that whilst there is no legislation stipulating an upper age limit for couples seeking IVF treatment, clinics who ultimately make a decision about whether or not to treat must act with care. The Authority does stipulate that there must be no harm to the child or parents through the use of IVF treatment and it is likely that there will be much further debate on the subject as further IVF babies are born to older mothers.

Desperate people may resort to desperate measures to avoid the guidelines some countries have in place. There are couples so keen to have children later in life that they have travelled abroad to undergo IVF after clinics in their home country had refused treatment. You can find clinics on the internet offering 'Holiday IVF' in some parts of Europe.

In every longed-for pregnancy there may be joy, but the abiding, ever-present need must be to consider the welfare of the child first, not the happiness of the parents. These days, parenthood spans at least twenty years, with many children still relying on their parents financially and emotionally well into their twenties. A lack of such assistance because of parents being in their eighties or nineties, frail and possibly suffering illness, can leave young people 'rudderless' and be a precursor to depression and anxiety. Such children, when reaching adulthood, may suffer severe emotional instability.

Technology is offering potential solutions to the problem of women being forced to leave motherhood beyond the traditional twenties and thirties. Clinics in America offer women in their twenties the chance to harvest their eggs while they are in good condition and plentiful. These eggs are frozen and stored for later use, perhaps when the woman finds a partner. Previously, unfertilised eggs were difficult to freeze successfully as the delicate structures of cells became badly damaged when thawed. New technology has enabled the freezing process to be achieved with far less damage.

Still, there remain limitations to this 'safe storage' option. Girls approaching the peak of their fertility in their late teens cannot yet afford to rely on egg storage technology if they want to guarantee they will experience motherhood. And research so far investigating IVF success for older women points to the fact that the rate of pregnancy for women over forty may be only half that of those aged thirty-five. The *Assisted Reproduction Report* for 2004, published by the US Centre for Disease Control, reveals less than 1 per cent of fresh cycles for women over forty-four resulted in a live birth.[3] Even good-quality donor embryos do not implant as successfully in women in their forties as they do in those under thirty.

Women may not be able to guarantee that they will conceive later in life, but a new test on the market is providing the opportunity for them to track their fertility levels and to be alerted if fertility drops rapidly. The test, called Plan Ahead, was developed by Professor Bill Ledger of Sheffield University. It measures hormone concentrations in the blood, which equate to an estimate of the number of eggs remaining in the ovaries. The test indicates fertility levels up to two years ahead; testing is recommended every few years. Other research is being undertaken on developing a blood test and high-quality ultrasound which, when taken together, may be a good indication of fertility.

Fertility tests are becoming a significant tool for older women to use to track fertility. The ability to plan parenthood with some certainty is highly appealing to many couples. Research over the next few years will determine just how accurate science can be in determining how many years of fertility a woman has left. Once this information is found to be reliable, couples can at least make more informed decisions about family planning, rather than attempting to conceive without being able to measure how likely they are to succeed.

What is a nuclear family?

IVF has also raised controversy about its ability to provide babies without a traditional biological mother and father. Fierce debate rages over the use of IVF for gay and lesbian couples and for single mothers. These three groups are seeking to define their rights to have children, the same rights available to heterosexual couples.

Technology is developing more rapidly than guidelines and laws can be put in place. Artificial insemination of a woman has been possible since before IVF came along; with lesbian couples, this technique excluded the partner of the mother from having a biological connection to the child. A more recent IVF technique known as intra-partner oocyte donation has changed this situation, now including both partners in the process.[4] One partner in a lesbian relationship donates the egg, which is artificially fertilised with donor sperm and implanted in the womb of the other female partner. The resulting baby then has a physical and emotional bond to both women.

For gay males in some countries there is an option to use a 'gestational carrier', a woman willing to be inseminated with one male partner's sperm and carry the baby until birth. IVF technology has gone one step further in allowing both male partners to contribute sperm, sometimes mixing this before fertilisation of the harvested egg from the gestational carrier. This method involves the participation of both partners in the process of conceiving their child.

Lesbian women are not excluded from treatment in some countries, though best practice in other countries recommends treatment is given only if the woman is medically infertile. The UK recently recognised same sex marriages and adoption by same sex couples and does not preclude lesbian women from seeking IVF treatment. Clinics are able to use their discretion in accepting couples for treatment assessing their suitability to care for a child and the strength of the relationship irrespective of sexual orientation.

British legislation has also enabled IVF treatment for single mothers. Again, it is the ability to financially and emotionally care for a child that is assessed rather than the nature of a relationship.

There is little research available that allows us to make informed decisions regarding different family scenarios and whether these are in the best interests of the children concerned. The few studies published appear to show no major differences for children raised in same-sex families versus traditional families. Children raised within same-sex relationships appear to do well emotionally and academically. Same-sex parents seem to be just as nurturing, organised and attentive as traditional parents. Same-sex parents are much more able to disclose the donor nature of their child's conception (they have little choice) and appear competent in ensuring children have access to both male and female role models. Small differences do appear to exist between children in same-sex families compared with those in traditional families. Small children of same-sex parents seem to engage in less gender-specific play, such as girls playing with dolls and boys with trucks, than small children with traditional parents. Teens raised by same-sex parents report more same-sex experiences than other teens. Differences also occur in the way children with same-sex parents are treated by others. They are more likely to be teased and bullied about their parents than children with heterosexual parents, a fact that can seriously undermine self-esteem.[5]

It is very worthwhile to consider how we can help same-sex parents requiring assistance to ensure their children are well balanced and happy. After all, this is no different to the manner in which we have long focused our efforts on trying to promote well-balanced and happy children parented by heterosexual couples and by single parents. We need to study and publish findings that promote the best same-sex parenting possible, as well as providing advice on how to help children cope with any negative reactions from peers about their same-sex parents.

Surrogacy

Surrogacy is another controversial issue involving IVF. A surrogacy arrangement is one in which a woman agrees to carry a foetus to term on behalf of another couple, known as the 'commissioning' parent(s). Generally, the surrogate mother is implanted with the commissioning couple's fertilised embryo using IVF. Once the baby is born, the surrogate mother hands over the baby.

There are a number of variations. The surrogate mother may have an embryo implanted that resulted from the commissioning father's sperm and the surrogate mother's egg. Occasionally, the surrogate mother may have an embryo implanted donated by another couple.

This arrangement has both biological and psychological consequences for the commissioning parents, the surrogate mother, her partner and the resulting child. The complexity of decisions around surrogacy stems from the number of people involved, the emotions stirred by pregnancy and birth, and by the lack of evidence about how families using this path to parenthood fare in the long term. It is also controversial because a baby conceived and carried using a surrogate mother may legally remain under the care of the surrogate mother and her partner, even though the embryo used to conceive through IVF may belong to the commissioning couple.

The media has consistently portrayed surrogacy as a somewhat 'underground' operation in which large sums of money are handed over and the people involved rarely keep their promises to each other. A widely publicised court case in 1998 produced heated debate after a one-year-old baby was removed from the commissioning parents to live with the mother who had acted as surrogate. This action was taken despite the fact that the sperm used to produce the baby was provided by the commissioning father. The surrogate mother's change of heart had both legal and public opinion heavily divided. For those involved, this must have been agonising, whatever the result handed down by the court.

Surrogacy is legal in the UK and in the US. In the UK, no money must be paid to the surrogate mother other than for the expenses incurred during pregnancy and birth. UK law does not recognise a surrogacy arrangement as legally binding until a parental order is obtained which may be granted six weeks after birth. Until such an order occurs, the surrogate mother has full rights over the baby she is carrying even if the baby was conceived using eggs and sperm from the commissioning couple. Once born, the commissioning father will have his name on the baby's birth certificate if his sperm was used and will have equal rights with the surrogate mother until parental orders are in place.

Surrogacy may be more widespread than statistics indicate. There is anonymously reported anecdotal evidence of parents donating embryos to other couples when, in reality, the couple receiving the donated embryo are acting as surrogates for the donating couple. The resulting baby may be later returned to the parents who donated the embryo. The consequences of this underground practice are very significant for all concerned. The secrecy necessary to achieve such a surrogacy arrangement means that during the pregnancy both surrogate and commissioning parents may be isolated from friends and family to avoid any person unwittingly discovering the secret. The child born as a result of such an arrangement may suffer psychological instability with the secrecy surrounding his conception and birth leading to feelings of not belonging. It may also be the case that arrangements which break down because of those involved changing their minds are not reported to authorities. In these situations, it is hard to ensure the well-being of the child who is caught up in such a contractual disaster.

Surrogacy, whether planned within legal guidelines or not, is fraught with difficulty, particularly if the child born is not the child that was expected or if the commissioning parents' situation changes. Babies are sometimes, although rarely, born with serious illnesses or abnormalities: it is hard to imagine how both the surrogate mother and the commissioning parents would feel about a baby with, for example, cerebral palsy. Would the commissioning parents change their minds? Would they be able to hold a surrogate mother financially liable for giving birth to a baby with an abnormality?

A further complication arises if the commissioning parents separate or if one dies during the pregnancy. If either scenario occurs, and the commissioning parents do not want to accept the child, would the surrogate mother feel compelled to keep the baby? Would the commissioning couple, after separation, launch a custody battle with each other, over a baby that another woman was carrying?

Although surrogacy can be a valid and psychologically beneficial option — for example, when a woman carries a baby for her infertile sibling — the laws governing the practice need to address all its complexities. Arrangements need to be formally agreed so that all parties know their rights. Most importantly, the child must be protected at all times. A baby who begins the first months of life with one set of parents needs to remain with them, even if there are disagreements between parties involved in the surrogacy. This is the only way to ensure the child develops a healthy and stable identity.

Testing

When IVF first became successful, doctors had little information about the qualities that made eggs, sperm and embryos 'better' or 'less likely to survive'. It was a far more random procedure in the 1980s to select eggs, fertilise them and implant one or two embryos than is the case in modern IVF treatment. Technological advances continue to transform the nature of the tests that can be performed in the laboratory, both before and after fertilisation.

Every year, scientists are identifying ever more characteristics that determine healthy eggs, better quality sperm and more 'successful' embryos. They are able to assess eggs and sperm, choosing the best to use for fertilisation and, later, testing the resulting embryos to rule out many of the genetic abnormalities that can affect the success of the pregnancy and the health of the resulting baby. This has brought about a better success rate for IVF treatment and a reduced incidence of birth defects. However, such advances also increase the possibilities for humankind to manipulate the world.

Now that we can genetically examine embryos, it is possible to determine the gender of these embryos and ultimately manipulate the natural distribution of males and females in the world. Already, IVF has disturbed the naturally occurring ratio of males to females. As a process, IVF requires the selection of the best quality embryos at day five after fertilisation. Since male embryos tend to divide faster than female embryos, rather more male embryos are implanted than females. The ratio of male to female babies born naturally is just over 51 per cent males to about 49 per cent females. IVF, however, results in around 58 per cent of male babies compared with 42 per cent of females. If the rate of IVF births continues to increase, we could see future generations in which it is much more difficult for men to find a mate.

We also have the power to pre-determine gender through IVF treatment with around 90 per cent certainty. One method is to only implant embryos of one gender. A second method is to sort sperm, since the two types — one carrying an X chromosome (female), the other a Y chromosome (male) — have different properties. Successful gender selection is not guaranteed, but the odds of producing one gender over the other are greatly enhanced.

Clearly, there are social and cultural implications involved in gender determination. As mentioned earlier, a preponderance of one gender over the other in one region or country could lead to serious social problems for adults who cannot find romantic partners. Culturally, there are already instances where a baby of one gender is more highly regarded than another. If IVF could produce the gender requested by parents for cultural reasons, it could also lead to serious shifts in the make-up of a society. In this instance, we are able to achieve scientific change that may not necessarily benefit us as a species.

The increasing ability of science to test embryos for genetic irregularities can also produce instances when babies are conceived and born specifically to help sick siblings. Generally, the baby is conceived through

IVF, the procedure enabling only embryos that are a genetic match to the sick child to be selected and implanted. Jodi Piccoult wrote a highly emotional novel about just such a scenario. In *My Sister's Keeper*, Piccoult describes the life led by a child conceived solely as a cure for her sister. It is compelling fiction and provides a highly informative window into the agonising decisions and complex emotions faced by families with a gravely sick child.

In the future, IVF may also offer the chance to screen embryos for life-threatening diseases such as cancer, heart disease and diabetes. This allows for the amazing possibility that IVF-conceived children will be healthier and live for longer than children conceived naturally. If it is possible to test for genetic illnesses, could we also in time be able to test for genetic characteristics, such as intelligence, sociability and personality? Or detect personality disorders that have genetic links? It is interesting to wonder how parents would feel if such complex genetic testing were available. Would fertile parents who have the financial means feel pressure to use IVF treatment and genetic screening to ensure their babies are as healthy physically and emotionally as those conceived by infertile couples through IVF? Indeed, would such testing make it unfashionable to conceive babies by natural means? It may be the case that the young children currently being raised may face such complex and emotional decisions by the time they are ready to be parents.

As well as these psychological and physical factors, the implications for the personal finances of those who may wish to use IVF and the overall costs to governments are considerable.

New directions

Other discoveries are creating a whole new world of infertility management that will overcome many fertility-diminishing factors. These discoveries are not likely to reduce the need for IVF but, instead, may help couples achieve pregnancy with greater success than if IVF were used alone.

Around one-third of infertile couples who turn to IVF do so because there are problems with the male partner's fertility. Dr Kelton Tremellen has developed a male fertility pill, called Menevit, which has already led to a doubling of the pregnancy rates of treated infertile couples. The pill blends antioxidants and minerals used to counteract the effects of smoking, environmental hazards and obesity. It is possible that such a treatment may be used for men who are contributing sperm to the IVF process to ensure that the sperm are of the best quality.

Major discoveries are also being made about the chemicals necessary for an embryo to successfully implant and develop inside a woman's womb. And we are learning about the factors that can inhibit implantation. Research is being undertaken to investigate certain gels that can be applied to make the womb a more welcoming place for embryos, which may arrive there either naturally or through assisted conception. Again, it is possible that such treatments may be used in conjunction with IVF to enhance success rates.

The success of IVF, and the amount of media attention given to it, has also led to a greater willingness by couples to accept fertility problems and to obtain treatment. Infertility is certainly not the 'black mark' it used to be, although there is still some way to go before this subject is casually discussed. Much greater amounts of research funding are being allocated to fertility treatment and a significantly higher profile is being given to those researchers who are successful in achieving increased rates of pregnancy. The intense media attention will ensure that fertility treatment is a vibrant area of research for many years to come.

Epilogue

By writing this book, my aim is to help anxious and stressed IVF parents enjoy the experience of parenting. I hope to ensure parents will be able to celebrate the wonderful journey that they have undertaken more easily. This enjoyment is extremely important. Parents need to feel they can be proud and happy to have achieved the miracle they have desired for so long.

Helping parents through IVF treatment, pregnancy and early parenting has been a much more emotional experience than I ever imagined it would be. There is such an instinctive and urgent need to conceive for couples who have been trying to have a baby for some time and, initially, I was unprepared to witness the pain generated by this unfulfilled need. Some of the parents I met had spent more than eight years trying IVF before eventually conceiving their children. The strength of the desire to have a baby is, at times, unimaginable to anyone who has not been denied this most fundamental human purpose, to reproduce. Providing support for these couples has required me to undertake the most intense and fulfilling work of my career.

IVF treatment has completely revolutionised the way we approach conception. Even for those couples who do not need to use the technique, the technology has provided a safeguard, a last resort they can turn to if their natural miracle does not occur. For other couples, the image of a bleak and childless future that came with a diagnosis of infertility has been replaced with joyous family scenes. To describe the technique as utterly remarkable is quite simply an understatement.

I sense, however, that professionals working in the sphere of fertility treatment have reached a crossroads in terms of the care they can provide for IVF couples. At first, IVF research centred solely on improving rates of success. The psychological issues for the couples involved in treatment were probably not even considered by these early research teams, when a successful pregnancy and healthy baby were thought to be the remedy for the grief couples may have felt before their treatment. This picture has changed considerably. So much of the recent research about IVF describes the intense and highly emotional transitions IVF parents are forced to make as they proceed through treatment. No longer do researchers confine themselves to describing the optimal chemicals, techniques and diagnostics that improve treatment options. Now, it is acknowledged that the psychological health of both partners is critical to the treatment process. New and exciting research is on the way that will give further weight to the role played by psychology in the process of conception. We will learn many new facts about how the mind and body work in unison to achieve implantation and embryo development.

I am fascinated by the possible future scenario of couples being prepared psychologically for IVF treatment as rigorously as they are now prepared physically. We may well conduct psychological therapy on specific days, using specific treatments, the way hormone injections and blood tests are used now. I believe we are only one step away from knowing that counselling needs to be provided before couples reach the stage of the first hormonal injection and on what day this would be best conducted. We are near to knowing that such therapies as acupuncture need to be performed on certain days before and after implantation to ensure success and that relaxation therapies such as massage during pregnancy ensure many more healthy, full-term babies than our conventional IVF approach to date.

Whatever the roles played by both biology and psychology in the process of conception, however, nothing will diminish the miracle that is IVF. Humankind never expected to be able to create new life within the confines of a glass tube. Now that we can, these tiny miracles, and their parents, deserve the very best care and support we can possibly provide them.

References

Introduction

1. McQuillan, J., Greil, A., White, L., Casey Jacob, M. (2003). Frustrated fertility: infertility and psychological distress among women. *Journal of Marriage and Family*, vol 65, no 4, pp 1007–18.

2. Peterson, B., Newton, C., Rosen, K., Skaggs, G. (2006). Gender differences in how men and women who are referred for IVF cope with infertility stress. *Human Reproduction*, vol 21, no 9, pp 2443–49.

3. Knoester, M., Helmerhorst, F., van der Westerlaken, L., Walther, F., Veen, S. (2007). Matched follow up study of 5-8 year old ICSI singletons. Human Reproduction vol. 22 (12), pp 3098-3017.

4. Ulrich, D., Gagel, D., Hemmerling, A., Pastor, V. (2004). Couples becoming parents: something special after IVF? Journal of Psychosomatic Obstetrics and Gynaecology, vol. 25 (2). pp 99-113.

Chapter One

1. Cook, R., Bradley, S., Golombok. (1998). A preliminary study of parental stress and child behaviour in families with twins conceived by in-vitro fertilisation. Human Reproduction, Vol 13, No. 11, pp 3244-3246.

2. Colpin, H., De Munter, A., Nys, K. (1999). Parenting stress and psychosocial wellbeing among parents with twins conceived naturally or by reproductive technology. Human Reproduction, Vol 14, No. 12, pp 3133-3137.

3. Peterson, b., Newton, C., Rosen, K., Schulman, R. (2006). Coping processes of couples experiencing infertility. Family Relations, Vol 55, No 2, pp227-39.

Chapter Two

1. Chavarro, J., Rich-Edwards, J., Rosner, B., Willett, W. (2007). Dietary fatty acid intakes and the risk of ovulatory infertility. *The American Journal of Clinical Nutrition*, vol 85, no 2, pp 231–37.

2. Campagne, D. (2006). Should fertilization treatment begin with reducing stress? *Human Reproduction*, vol 21, no 7, pp 1651–58.

3. Smith, C., Coyle, M., Norman, R. (2006). Influence of acupuncture stimulation on pregnancy rates for women undergoing embryo transfer. *Fertility and Sterility*, vol 85, no 5, pp 1352–58.

4. Levitas, E., Parmet, A., Lunenfield, E., *et al.* (2006). Impact of hypnosis during embryo transfer on the outcome of in vitro fertilization embryo transfer: a case control study. *Fertility and Sterility*, vol 85, no 5, pp 1404–08.

Chapter Three

1. Pelinck, M., Vogel, N., Hoek, A., *et al.* (2006). Cumulative pregnancy rates after three cycles of minimal stimulation IVF and results according to subfertility diagnosis: a multicentre cohort study. *Human Reproduction*, vol 21, no 9, pp 2375–83.

2. Pistorious, E., Adang, E., Stalmeier, P., *et al.* (2006). Prospective patient and physician preferences for stimulation or no stimulation in IVF. *Human Fertility*, vol 9, no 4, pp 209–16.

3. Child, T.J., Phillips, S.J., Abdul-Jalil, A.K., *et al.* (2002). A comparison of in vitro maturation and in vitro fertilisation for women with polycystic ovaries. *Obstetrics and Gynaecology*, vol 100, pp 665–70.

4. Svanberg, A., Boivin, J., Hjelmstedt, A., *et al.* (2001). The impact of frozen embryos on emotional reactions during in vitro fertilisation. *Obstetrica et Gynecologica Scandinavica*, vol 80, no 12, pp 1110–14.

5. Applegarth, L. (2003). Donor options: egg, sperm and embryo. Available at www.webmd.com/content/article/74/89195.htm.

6. Verhaak, C., Smeenk, J., Evers, A., *et al.* (2005). Predicting emotional response to unsuccessful fertility treatment. *Journal of Behavioural Medicine*, vol 28, no 2, pp 181–90.

7. Olivius, K., Friden, B., Lundin, K., Bergh, C. (2002). Cumulative probability of live birth after three in vitro fertilisation/intracytoplasmic sperm injection cycles. *Fertility and Sterility*, vol 77, no 3, pp 505–10.

Chapter Four

1. Kennedy, R. (2006). Ricks and complications of assisted conception. British Fertility Society factsheet, available at www.britishfertilitysociety.org.uk/public/factsheets/keyfacts.html.

2. Eddleman, K. (2006). Is the risk of amniocentesis overrated? *Obstetrics and Gynecology*, vol 108, November, pp 1067–72.

3. Woldringh, G., Frunt, M., Kremer, J., Spaanderman, M. (2006). Decreased ovarian reserve relates to pre-eclampsia in IVF/ICSI pregnancies. *Human Reproduction*, vol 21, no 11, pp 2948–54.

4. Kallen, B., Finnstrom, O., Nygren, K., *et al.* (2005). In vitro fertilisation in Sweden: obstetric characteristics, maternal morbidity and mortality. *British Journal of Obstetrics and Gynaecology*, vol 112, no 11, pp 1529–35.

5. Field, T., Hernandez-Reif, M., Diego, M., *et al.* (2005). Cortisol decreases and serotonin and dopamine increase following pregnancy massage. *International Journal of Neuroscience*, vol 115, no 10, pp 1397–1413.

6. Field, T., Hernandez-Reif, M., Hart, S., *et al.* (1999). Pregnant women benefit from massage therapy. *Journal of Psychosomatic Obstetrics and Gynaecology*, vol 19, pp 31–38.

Chapter Five

1. Cyna, A., McAuliffe, G., Andrew, M. (2004). Hypnosis for pain relief in labour and childbirth: a systematic review. *British Journal of Anaesthesia*, vol 93, no 4, pp 505–11.

2. Scwartz, F. (1997). Music and perinatal stress reduction. *Journal of Prenatal and Perinatal Psychology*, vol 12, no 1, pp 19–30.

Chapter Six

1. Bornstein, M. (2002). The Handbook of Parenting, New Jersey: Lawrence Erlbaum and Associates.
2. Brazelton, B.T. (2006). Touchpoints: Birth to Three, 2nd edition, New York: Merloyd Lawrence.
3. Champion, H. (2006). The Baby Champion DVD, Australia: The Ussher Direction Pty Ltd.

Chapter Seven

1. Williamson, V. (2005). Unpublished PhD thesis. Available at www.adelaide. edu.au/news/news5586.html.
2. Sims, M., Guilfoyle, A., Parry, T. (2006). Childcare for infants and toddlers: where in the world are we going? *New Zealand Journal of Infant and Toddler Education*, vol 8, no 1, pp 12–19.
3. Colpin, H., De Munter, A., Nys, K. (1999). Parenting stress and psychosocial well-being among parents with twins conceived naturally or by reproductive technology. *Human Reproduction*, vol 14, no 12, pp 3133–37.
4. Munro, J., Ironside, W., Smith, G. (1992). Successful parents of in vitro fertilization: the social repercussions. *Journal of Assisted Reproductive Genetics*, vol 9, no 2, pp 170–76.

Chapter Eight

1. McNair, R. (2004). Outcomes for children born of assisted reproductive technology in a diverse range of families. Melbourne: Victorian Law Reform Commission, available at www.lawreform.vic.gov.au.
2. Grimm, N., (2006). IVF youth experiencing genetic anger. Australian Broadcasting Corporation, *7.30 Report*, 23 November 2006, available at www. abc.net.au/7.30/content/2006/s1796095.htm.
3. Daniels, K. (2004). New Zealand: from secrecy and shame to openness and acceptance. In Blythe, E., Landau, R. (eds) *Third-party Assisted Conception Across Cultures: Social, legal and ethical perspectives*. London: Jessica Kingsley.
4. Lycett, E., Daniels, K., Curson, R., Golombook, S. (2005). School-aged children

of donor insemination: a study of parents' disclosure patterns. *Human Reproduction*, vol 20, no 3, pp 810–19.

5. Rumball, A. (1999). Ethics and society: telling the story: parents' scripts for donor offspring. *Human Reproduction*, vol 14, no 5, pp 1392–99.

6. Murray, C., Golombok, S. (2003). To tell or not to tell: The decision-making process of egg donation parents. *Human Fertility*, vol 6, no 2, pp 89–95.

7. Schneller, E. (2005). The rights of donor inseminated children to know their genetic origins in Australia. *Australian Journal of Family Law*, vol 19, no 3, pp 222–44.

Chapter Nine

1. Lopez Teijon, M., Serra, O., Olivares, R., *et al.* (2006). Delivery of a healthy baby following the transfer of embryos cryopreserved for 13 years. *Reproduction*, vol 13, no 6, pp 821–22.

2. Kovacs, G., Breheny, S., Dear, M. (2003). Embryo donation at an Australian university in-vitro fertilisation clinic: issues and outcomes. *Medical Journal of Australia*, vol 178, no 3, pp 127–29.

3. Centres for Disease Control and Prevention (2004). *2004 Assisted Reproductive Report*. Available at www.cdc.gov.

4. Woodward, B., Norton, W. (2006). Lesbian intra-partner oocyte donation: a possible shake-up in the Garden of Eden? *Human Fertility*, vol 9, no 4, pp 217–22.

5. McNair, R. (2004). Outcomes for children born of assisted reproductive technology in a diverse range of families. Melbourne: Victorian Law Reform Commission, available at www.lawreform.vic.gov.au.

Useful Contacts

AMERICAN SOCIETY OF REPRODUCTIVE MEDICINE
Information about IVF treatment, reproductive specialists and the location of clinics in the US.
www.asrm.org

CHILDLESSNESS OVERCOME THROUGH SURROGACY (COTS)
UK support organisation for would-be parents and surrogates.
www.surrogacy.org.uk
Phone: 0844 414181

DONOR CONCEPTION NETWORK
A British-based organisation providing online information and booklets for parents of donor-conceived children.
www.dcnetwork.org
Postal address; PO Box 7471, Nottingham, UK.

DOULAS

To find out more about the services provided by doulas or to find a UK-based practitioner, visit:

www.doula.org.uk

EUROPEAN SOCIETY OF HUMAN REPRODUCTION (ESHRE)

Provides statistics of IVF treatment worldwide in addition to European legislation and best practice guidelines.

www.eshre.com

HUMAN FERTILISATION AND EMBRYOLOGY AUTHORITY

The UK's IVF regulator and a source of information on treatment, clinics, legislation and best practice guidelines.

www.hfea.gov.uk

IVF-INFERTILITY

A site designed by UK infertility specialists providing information about infertility, treatment and clinic details.

www.ivf-infertility.com

MOTHERS OVER FORTY

A British-based organisation providing online information and support to women who become mothers after the age of forty.

www.mothersover40.com

THE MULTIPLE BIRTHS FOUNDATION

An independent UK charity. A resource for professionals and families alike, aiming to improve the care and support of multiple birth families.

www.multiplebirths.org.uk

SANDS

SANDS provides bereavement information and support for parents and families who have suffered miscarriage or the loss of a baby in infancy.
www.uk-sands.org

X, Y AND ME

The website of nurse and author Janice Grimes who has written a series of books for IVF children explaining their genetic origins.
www.xyandme.com

Index

THE QUEST FOR A CHILD

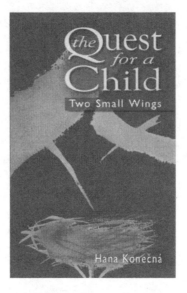

Hana Konečná

Faculty of Health and Social Studies, University of South Bohemia, Czech Republic

This book has been written to provide hope, support and information to couples trying to conceive a child. It evolved from research involving hundreds of childless couples, their doctors, and fertility specialists.

Written in a positive, empathetic and easy style, this book should bring comfort to anyone who is going through the pain of childlessness. It will also be valued by medical practitioners, social workers and allied health professionals who deal with childlessness in their daily work.

Price £14.99

ISBN 978 1 905740 772

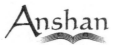